Complete Review for the Pharmacy Technician

Notices

SECOND EDITION

Complete Review for the Pharmacy Technician

L. MICHAEL POSEY, BPHARM

Editorial Director, Periodicals

American Pharmacists Association

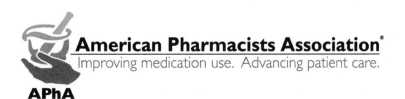

American Pharmacists Association®
Improving medication use. Advancing patient care.
APhA

Washington, D.C.

ACQUIRING EDITOR:
Sandra J. Cannon

SENIOR PROJECT MANAGER:
Vicki Meade, *Meade Communications*

MANAGING EDITOR:
Paula Novash

GRAPHIC DESIGNER:
Chris Borges, *Borges Creative*
Janette Lockhart

COVER DESIGN:
Scott Neitzke, *APhA Creative Services*

ILLUSTRATIONS:
Walter Hilmers Jr.

PHOTOGRAPHERS:
Janet Little (*pages 111-16, 128, 130-1, 134, 145, 150-1, 187-8, 194-5, 203*)
Philip Rink Jr. (*pages 112, 117, 134, 165, 168, 209*)

PROOFREADERS:
Amy Morgante
Mary DeAngelo

INDEXER:
Mary Coe

© 2007 by the American Pharmacists Association

Published by the American Pharmacists Association
1100 15th Street, NW, Suite 400
Washington, DC 20005-1707
www.pharmacist.com

APhA was founded in 1852 as the American Pharmaceutical Association

To comment on this book via e-mail, send your message to the publisher at
aphabooks@aphanet.org

LIBRARY OF CONGRESS CATALOGING-IN-PUBLICATION DATA

Posey, L. Michael.
    Complete review for the pharmacy technician / L. Michael Posey. -- 2nd ed.
        p. ; cm.
    Rev. ed. of: APhA's complete review for the pharmacy technician. 2001.
    Includes bibliographical references and index.
    ISBN 978-1-58212-094-2
    1. Pharmacy technicians. I. Posey, L. Michael. APhA's complete review
for the pharmacy technician. II. American Pharmacists Association. III.
Title.
        [DNLM: 1. Pharmacists' Aides. 2. Medication Systems, Hospital. 3.
Pharmaceutical Services. QV 21.5 P855a 2007]

RS122.95.P675 2007
615'.1--dc22   2007025760

HOW TO ORDER THIS BOOK

ONLINE:
www.pharmacist.com
VISA®, MasterCard®, and American Express® cards accepted.

BY PHONE:
800-878-0729
(from the United States and Canada)

Table of Contents

PART I

Basic Information

CHAPTER ONE
Role of the Pharmacy Technician in Pharmacy Practice
Shift of Pharmacists Away from Drug Preparation; Move Toward Clinical Pharmacy and Pharmaceutical Care; Need for a Paraprofessional in Pharmacy; Pharmacy Technicians Today

CHAPTER TWO
Pharmacy Calculations, Abbreviations, and Terminology
Pharmacy Calculations; Pharmaceutical Abbreviations; Medical Terminology

CHAPTER THREE
Pharmacy Governance
Food and Drug Administration; Centers for Medicare and Medicaid Services; Drug Enforcement Administration; Federal Patient Information Initiatives; State Boards of Pharmacy; Conditions for Participation and Accreditation Programs; Voluntary Accreditation and Certification Programs; Material Safety Data Sheets; Codes of Ethics

CHAPTER FOUR
Drug Classifications and Formulations
Normal Human Anatomy and Body Function; Pathophysiology: When Something is Wrong; Pharmacotherapy: Treating Disease with Drugs; Drug Interactions

PART II

Prescription Dispensing

PART III

Maintaining Medication and Inventory Control Systems

PART IV

Assisting with Pharmacy Administration and Management

Foreword

As a pharmacist, I know the positive impact that highly skilled and competent pharmacy technicians have had on my ability to deliver quality patient care in all the pharmacy practice settings in which I have been employed. Conversely, I am also aware of the difficulty in providing a high level of care when the pharmacy technician has not achieved an appropriate level of proficiency, either educationally or professionally.

For more than 40 years, the profession has engaged in debates addressing concerns, challenges and solutions focused on the training, utilization and recognition of pharmacy technicians in the practice of pharmacy.[1-2] Consistently, the call for a set of uniform technician education, training and competency standards, including a formalized, standard core, has emerged. One notable response to this need was the development and release of the Model Curriculum for Pharmacy Technician Training by the American Society of Health-System Pharmacists (ASHP) (1st ed: 1996; 2nd ed: 2001).[3] Pharmacy technician training program accreditation (e.g., ASHP), pharmacy technician continuing education (e.g., Accreditation Council on Pharmacy Education [ACPE]), national voluntary certification (e.g., Pharmacy Technician Certification Board [PTCB]; established 1995) and more regulation of technician activities (e.g., state board of pharmacy practice act revisions) have also been strongly supported. Why are these milestones important?

With the tremendous broadening of the pharmacist's role and responsibilities in providing patient-centered care (previously referred to as pharmaceutical care), increasingly, functions deemed as not requiring the pharmacist's "clinical judgment" are being performed by pharmacy technicians.[4] The increased use of pharmacy technicians has been recognized to have a substantial impact, both positively and negatively, on the efficiency and quality of services provided by the pharmacy care team.[5]

All pharmacy technicians should be used in the most effective and appropriate way to preserve public health and safety while minimizing medication-related risk. This can be accomplished through synergistic applications of knowledge, skills, abilities, and roles for pharmacists and technicians. All sectors of the profession should work collaboratively to ensure that technicians possess the knowledge, skills, and training necessary to accept these expanded roles. The scope of responsibilities delegated to pharmacy technicians should not be broadened until educational needs are satisfactorily addressed. Particularly, in light of recent negative media coverage suggesting diminishing professional standards pertaining to technician utilization (e.g., ABC News 20/20; April 3, 2007)[6], can we afford not to do so?

The importance of baseline core knowledge and skills for all pharmacy technicians cannot be overemphasized. This is a key elemental step in the formal and informal education process. This new edition of the *Complete Review for the Pharmacy Technician* embraces this philosophy by providing an initial learning tool for the neophyte as well as a review for the more experienced technician.

I hope that pharmacy technicians who use this reference will find it a valuable resource to help strengthen their knowledge, skill development, and professional commitment to work together with pharmacists to improve the lives and overall health of the patients we serve. We owe them nothing less.

Miriam A. Mobley Smith, *BPharm, PharmD*
Associate Professor and Chair
Department of Pharmacy Practice
College of Pharmacy
Chicago State University
July 2007

1. Sesquicentennial Stepping Stone Summits—Summit Two: Pharmacy Technicians. *J Am Pharm Assoc.* 2003;43:84-92.

2. White paper on pharmacy technicians (2002): needed changes can no longer wait. *J Am Pharm Assoc.* 2003;43:93-107.

3. American Society of Health-System Pharmacists. Model curriculum for pharmacy technician training. http://www.ashp.org/s_ashp/quart2c.asp?CID=3608&DID=5743 (accessed 2007 June 11).

4. Muenzen PM, Corrigan MM, Mobley Smith MA, Rodrigue PG. Updating the Pharmacy Technician Certification Examination: a practice analysis study. *Am J Health-Syst Pharm.* 2005;62:2542-6.

5. Weber EW, Hepfinger C, Koontz R, Cohn-Oswald L. Pharmacy technicians supporting clinical functions. *Am J Health-Syst Pharm.* 2005;62:2466,2469, 2472.

6. Pharmacy Errors: Unreported Epidemic? http://abcnews.go.com/video/playerIndex?id=2997449 (accessed 2007 June 11).

Preface to the Second Edition

Since this book was first published in 2001, pharmacies have experienced ever-increasing demands for a wider variety of services. Historically valued for the ability to prepare drug preparations, pharmacists are now depended upon for knowledge about powerful medications and the best ways to use them. The explosion of new drugs and information, plus the need for pharmaceutical care services and other responsibilities associated with Medicare Part D, means that pharmacists need paraprofessionals to help with the daily tasks involved in pharmacies now more than ever. This book seeks to provide information and support for those invaluable assistants, pharmacy technicians.

Like the first edition, the updated *Complete Review for the Pharmacy Technician* provides baseline knowledge for new community and health-system pharmacy technicians who are beginning in-house or on-the-job training, an introduction to the field for students entering formal technician-training programs, and concise review that can fill in gaps for pharmacy technicians with more experience. In addition, the text covers basic information needed to understand the Responsibilities and Knowledge that the Pharmacy Technician Certification Board (PTCB) tests for in its national examination. Based on the most recent Content Outline of the PTCB, these chapters cover every subject area and also list additional sources such as specialized APhA texts for further study.

This second edition also contains a wide range of new features that enhance the text and make it reader friendly: color illustrations and figures make the content more accessible, supplemental forms and tables collect important information for easy reference, and calculation exercises reinforce learning and encourage students to practice skills. The Appendix section refers students to areas in the book that correspond to the information covered in the PTCB Examination.

It is easy to envision a day when most of pharmacists' time is taken up by clinical duties and direct patient care. It is technicians who will keep the drug-distribution machinery running. Within this scenario, pharmacists and technicians must keep ever before them the needs of the patients they serve. Pharmacists' clinical roles serve little purpose if the right drug is not delivered to the right patient at the right time, and the best drug-delivery system is of little use if the medications are not used properly and in the correct doses in the treatment of human disease. Therefore, pharmacists and technicians must work together to ensure their patients' health and their own future in our rapidly evolving health care system. I hope this book contributes to their collaboration.

For their assistance in updating this manual and making it more useful to pharmacy technicians, I would like to thank Julian Graubart, Sandy Cannon and Kathy Anderson at APhA, as well as Vicki Meade and Paula Novash for their editorial services. I also appreciate the hospitality and forbearance of David A. Kotzin, RPh, BS, MS of the Terrapin Pharmacy, and Jay G. Barbaccia, PharmD, FASHP, Pharmacy Director, and the pharmacy staff at Washington Hospital Center, for graciously hosting us in their facilities and allowing us to photograph them for this book.

L. MICHAEL POSEY, *BPharm*
Athens, Georgia
June 2007

Acknowledgments

The author and publisher gratefully acknowledge the following individuals who assisted in the development of this second edition:

LAUREN ANGELO, *PharmD, MBA, Senior Manager, APhA Education Programs,* for assistance with the Medicare Part D and medication therapy management sections of Chapter 3, Pharmacy Governance.

KAREN SNIPE, *MAEd, CPhT, of Trident Technical College, Charleston, S.C.,* for sharing photographs for use in Chapter 10, Sterile Compounding and Radiopharmaceuticals.

KELLY WOLFE, *PharmD, of Muncie, Ind.,* for adding recently approved medications to the drugs table in Chapter 4, Drug Classifications and Formulations, and for adding structure to its adverse effects listings.

Basic Information

CHAPTER ONE

Role of the Pharmacy Technician in Pharmacy Practice

In this introductory chapter you will learn about the most common activities and responsibilities of the pharmacy technician practicing in the first decade of the 21st century. It reviews current trends in practice and describes the emergence of the pharmacy technician as an important part of contemporary pharmacy practice, including the development of pharmaceutical care, the economic and governmental pressures on pharmacy, and the increasing automation of the dispensing function formerly handled primarily by registered pharmacists.

The clinical pharmacy movement sought to create a role for pharmacists who would provide patient-specific drug information or advice to physicians and other members of the health care team.

Introduction

While pharmacists have long employed assistants to help in many aspects of prescription preparation and pharmacy operation, pharmacy technicians emerged quickly in the latter half of the 20th century as critically important to both the current development and the future prospects of the pharmacy profession. In the United States since 1980, the roles and responsibilities of pharmacy technicians have been delineated, and mechanisms for ensuring a minimum level of competency have been developed. Here we discuss the trends in pharmacy that are accelerating the need for and use of technicians.

Shift of Pharmacists Away from Drug Preparation

Pharmacy—sometimes referred to as the world's second oldest profession—has been around for literally thousands of years. In recorded history, the earliest mentions of people who specialized in the use of plants and herbal products were in ancient Babylon and China, both at about 2000 BC.

For most of the intervening 4000 years, pharmacists have been largely concerned with the mechanical preparation of medicines for specific patients. Patients needed pharmacists to incorporate medicinal products into gargles, snuffs, inhalations, suppositories, fumigations, enemas, poultices, decoctions, infusions, pills, troches, lotions, ointments, and plasters. Often of plant origin, such products were of limited effectiveness, but they were all that was available for most of recorded history.

However, with the rapid advances in scientific knowledge over the past three centuries, much progress was made in developing effective and safe drugs. In the late 1930s and early 1940s, anti-infective drugs became available that made a remarkable difference in survival rates of soldiers during World War II. That is, soldiers wounded in battle who would have died in earlier wars from infections were cured using miracle drugs such as penicillin.

The availability of these drugs fueled a rapid growth in the *pharmaceutical industry* (the companies that manufacture and distribute medications, such as GlaxoSmithKline, Novartis, sanofi aventis, Merck, and Lilly) during and after World War II. As a result, the kind of work that pharmacists performed suddenly shifted from preparing drug products (*compounding*) to *dispensing* commercially available products (sometimes disparagingly called "counting, pouring, licking, and sticking"). Pharmacists found themselves suddenly short on professional esteem, a trend that perhaps reached a low point in 1975 when one Supreme Court Justice wrote in an opinion that a pharmacist was no more a professional than a clerk who sold law books.

Move Toward Clinical Pharmacy and Pharmaceutical Care

In the late 1950s and 1960s, astute pharmacists such as Donald C. Brodie of the University of California–San Francisco, Donald E. Francke of the University of Michigan, and Paul F. Parker of the University of Kentucky began to dream of a new role for pharmacists that would involve the specialized provision of information about the powerful new agents that were becoming available from the pharmaceutical industry. The *clinical pharmacy movement*, as it came to be known, sought to create a role for pharmacists who would provide patient-specific drug information or advice to physicians and other members of the health care team.

Clinical pharmacy, which began primarily in large teaching hospitals, grew out of a need for advanced, detailed, and interpretive drug information combined with drug-distribution programs in hospitals, which, in turn, moved pharmacists out of the central pharmacy and onto patient-care units. Beginning in 1966 with pilot programs at University of California–San Francisco, the clinical pharmacy movement soon was adopted to varying degrees in schools of pharmacy and in most US teaching hospital pharmacies.

In the late 1980s, two other pharmacy visionaries—Charles D. Hepler and Linda M. Strand, who were both at the University of Florida at the time—began to describe ways the ideals, goals, and functions of the clinical pharmacy movement could be translated into all areas of pharmacy practice. Soon dubbed *pharmaceutical care*, this view of pharmacy practice maintained that all pharmacists—regardless of where they worked—should deliver the same kind of care using a standard process that would most likely result in improvements in patients' health. The definition of pharmaceutical care is provided in Chapter 6, where it is discussed in detail.

By 1990, other trends were evident that would further drive the pharmacists into more "cognitive" roles in patient care. First, the American Council on Pharmaceutical Education announced its intention to phase out the bachelor of science in pharmacy degree in favor of a "new" *doctor of pharmacy* degree. With the last of the BS degree programs going out of existence in 2004, this change means that all pharmacists will enter the profession with an extra year of training, mostly in clinical and disease-management areas.

The second trend was a new requirement mandated by the US Congress. In passing the Omnibus Budget Reconciliation Act (OBRA) of 1990, Congress required pharmacists to offer to counsel and review the drug regimens of people in the Medicaid program. OBRA '90, which was rapidly enacted for all patients by most state boards of pharmacy, gave new life to the hope that pharmacists would be able to reprofessionalize themselves and keep their profession alive into the 21st century.

As described in Chapter 3, these trends have now led to creation of a medication therapy management benefit under the recently enacted drug benefit for Medicare patients. These elderly and disabled individuals now have access to a federally funded program in which pharmacists and other qualified health professionals can be compensated for assisting with complicated, expensive drug regimens.

Need for a Paraprofessional in Pharmacy

As these events unfolded, pharmacists quickly realized that they could not spend the majority of their time "counting, pouring, licking, and sticking" and still be able to take advantage of the opportunities for advancing pharmacy practice. Beginning in the 1950s and 1960s, hospitals were the first to incorporate an identifiable group of *pharmacy assistants* into daily operations. Pharmacists found themselves freed to go on rounds with physicians and medical residents because well-trained technicians could keep the pharmacy running in their absence.

The US military also incorporated pharmacy assistants into practice. Well-designed military training programs produced knowledgeable pharmacy assistants. Because the military operates outside state law, pharmacists were free to use pharmacy assistants creatively as they became widely available within the Army, Navy, and Air Force.

During the 1980s, pharmacy struggled to determine appropriate ways to train and recognize pharmacy technicians, who were generally called *pharmacy support personnel*. While national groups tended to believe that technicians should be trained formally in community colleges or technical schools, the reality was that most were simply high school graduates who had been trained on the job in community or hospital pharmacies.

Two state groups recognized this disparity. First the Michigan Pharmacists Association (MPA) and later the Illinois Council of Hospital (now Health-System) Pharmacists (ICHP) independently developed *certification examinations for pharmacy technicians*. These voluntary programs involved written examinations that sought to recognize a minimum level of knowledge thought to be needed by those working as pharmacy technicians. The examinations were so successful in Michigan and Illinois that both groups began marketing their

Pharmacy technicians are a diverse lot, ranging from career employees who have worked for decades in this field to student pharmacists who are employed in this capacity while they pursue a pharmacy degree.

FIGURE 1-1

Number of Certified Pharmacy Technicians Recognized by the Pharmacy Technician Certification Board, by State, as of March 31, 2007.

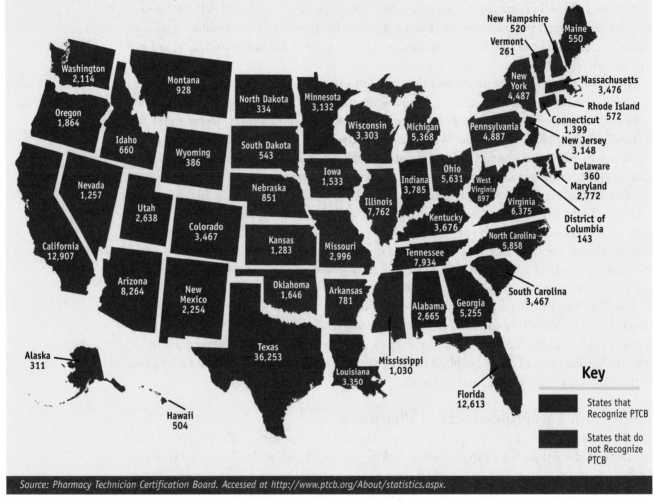

Washington 2,114
Montana 928
North Dakota 334
Minnesota 3,132
New Hampshire 520
Vermont 261
Maine 550
New York 4,487
Massachusetts 3,476
Rhode Island 572
Oregon 1,864
Idaho 660
Wyoming 386
South Dakota 543
Wisconsin 3,303
Michigan 5,368
Pennsylvania 4,887
Connecticut 1,399
New Jersey 3,148
Nevada 1,257
Utah 2,638
Nebraska 851
Iowa 1,533
Indiana 3,785
Ohio 5,631
West Virginia 897
Delaware 360
Maryland 2,772
California 12,907
Colorado 3,467
Kansas 1,283
Missouri 2,996
Illinois 7,762
Kentucky 3,676
Virginia 6,375
District of Columbia 143
North Carolina 5,858
Arizona 8,264
New Mexico 2,254
Oklahoma 1,646
Arkansas 781
Tennessee 7,934
Alabama 2,665
Georgia 5,255
South Carolina 3,467
Alaska 311
Texas 36,253
Mississippi 1,030
Louisiana 3,350
Florida 12,613
Hawaii 504

Key

States that Recognize PTCB

States that do not Recognize PTCB

Source: Pharmacy Technician Certification Board. Accessed at http://www.ptcb.org/About/statistics.aspx.

certification processes to other state organizations. By the mid-1990s, more than one half of the states in the United States were offering either the Michigan or the Illinois examination to pharmacy technicians.

As pharmacists increasingly saw the benefit of formally assessing the knowledge of those who assisted them in prescription dispensing, the American Pharmaceutical (now Pharmacists) Association and the American Society of Health-System Pharmacists joined with MPA and ICHP to form the Pharmacy Technician Certification Board (PTCB), which now administers a single national exam. Since its inception in 1995, more than 250,000 *Certified Pharmacy Technicians* (CPhTs) have been recognized by either meeting the national requirements or by continuing their certification obtained previously under the Michigan or Illinois examination. States have increasingly incorporated registration of technicians into pharmacy practice laws, and many states also now recognize national certification as a requirement for working as a pharmacy technician or to perform certain tasks (see Figure 1-1). The availability of such a large group of recognized paraprofessionals who can assist in preparing and dispensing prescriptions promises to enable pharmacists to further develop their pharmaceutical care and medication therapy management services.

Pharmacy Technicians Today

Pharmacy technicians are a diverse lot, ranging from career employees who have worked for decades in this field to student pharmacists who are employed in this capacity while they pursue a pharmacy degree. A 2004 survey[1] showed that nearly 90% of 965 CPhTs were employed in either chain or independent community pharmacy or hospital pharmacy (Figure 1-2). The average wage at that time was $12.87 per hour; for the 10.7% of CPhTs who were members of unions, this figure was $14.70.

Job satisfaction was also explored in this survey. Overall, CPhTs were moderately satisfied with their current positions although they were somewhat less committed to the current employers than other surveys have shown pharmacists to be. On-the-job stressors for CPhTs were "inadequate staffing" and "other technicians not doing their jobs properly."[2]

A further analysis of these 2004 data showed that about 80% of CPhTs intended to remain with their current employer during the next 12 months. CPhTs cited relationships with coworkers, good benefits, and work schedule as reasons to remain in the current jobs, and they pointed to these factors as reasons to move on: poor salary, lack of advancement opportunity, and insufficient staffing.[3]

FIGURE 1-2

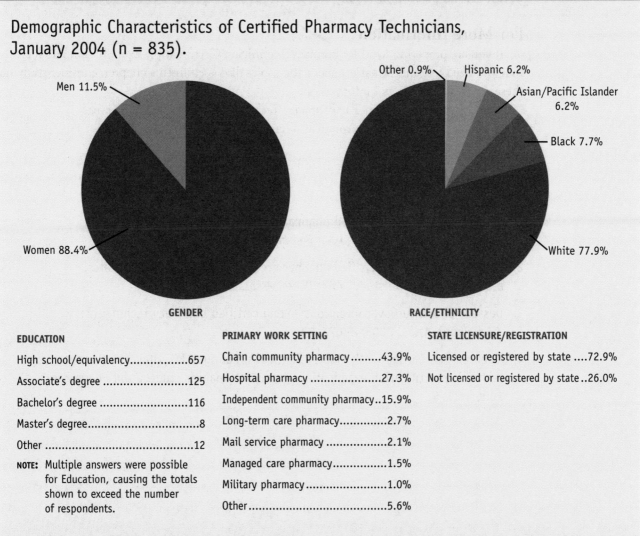

Demographic Characteristics of Certified Pharmacy Technicians, January 2004 (n = 835).

Men 11.5%
Women 88.4%

GENDER

Other 0.9%
Hispanic 6.2%
Asian/Pacific Islander 6.2%
Black 7.7%
White 77.9%

RACE/ETHNICITY

EDUCATION

High school/equivalency.................657

Associate's degree 125

Bachelor's degree 116

Master's degree.................................8

Other 12

NOTE: Multiple answers were possible for Education, causing the totals shown to exceed the number of respondents.

PRIMARY WORK SETTING

Chain community pharmacy.........43.9%

Hospital pharmacy 27.3%

Independent community pharmacy..15.9%

Long-term care pharmacy.............2.7%

Mail service pharmacy 2.1%

Managed care pharmacy...............1.5%

Military pharmacy 1.0%

Other...5.6%

STATE LICENSURE/REGISTRATION

Licensed or registered by state 72.9%

Not licensed or registered by state ..26.0%

Source: Desselle S. Survey of certified pharmacy technicians in the United States: a quality-of-worklife study. J Am Pharm Assoc. 2005;45:458-65.

In a 2005 survey conducted by the PTCB, 1,040 CPhTs provided several noteworthy pieces of information[4]:

- On average, CPhTs were spending 63% of their time assisting the pharmacist in serving patients, 23% maintaining medication and inventory control systems, and 14% helping with pharmacy management and administration. These percentages have been adopted by PTCB on the certification examinations now being administered (see the Appendices for the specific knowledge and responsibility statements that PTCB uses in constructing the examination and on which the content of this book is based).
- Formal on-the-job training had been provided to 40% of CPhTs, an increase over the 29% with this type of training in a similar 1999 survey.
- The percentage of CPhTs with supervisory responsibilities had increased to 40% from 32% in 1999.

To ensure your success as a pharmacy technician, the remaining chapters in this book provide an overview of and basic information about the topics most relevant to your daily activities. While you need to learn many facts to properly and safely assist with the practice of pharmacy, your position as a pharmacy technician can offer you a lifetime of satisfying and rewarding experiences as you support the activities of the world's second oldest profession.

For More Information

If you are preparing for the Pharmacy Technician Certification Examination and feel that you need more information about the topics discussed in this chapter, consider studying these sources of additional information:

- Chapters 2 and 3 in *The Pharmacy Technician's Introduction to Pharmacy*, by L. Michael Posey. American Pharmacists Association. 2007 (in press).
- Read the journal articles listed below as references.

References

1. Desselle S. Survey of certified pharmacy technicians in the United States: a quality-of-worklife study. *J Am Pharm Assoc.* 2005; 45:458-65.

2. Desselle S. Survey of certified pharmacy technicians in the United States: a quality-of-worklife study. *J Am Pharm Assoc.* 2005; 45:458-65.

3. Desselle S. Job turnover intentions among certified pharmacy technicians. *J Am Pharm Assoc.* 2005;45:676–83.

4. Muenzen PM, Corrigan MM, Mobley Smith MA, Rodrigue PG. Updating the pharmacy technician certification examination: a practice analysis study. *J Am Pharm Assoc.* 2006;46:1–6.

CHAPTER TWO

Pharmacy Calculations, Abbreviations, and Terminology

Chapter 2 presents information in three key areas of knowledge. First it shows calculations as a mixture of straightforward explanations and practical problems. Next it presents abbreviations, primarily in a table, with a brief explanation of their Latin origins. Then it discusses commonly used medical terminology in list form, again with a brief description of word origins and roots.

Introduction

The next three chapters provide basic information that you will need when we get to the heart of this book, Chapter 5, which covers the processing of prescriptions. In this chapter, you'll learn about pharmacy calculations, medical terminology, and abbreviations used in pharmacy and by doctors when they write prescriptions and other types of medication orders.

Pharmacy Calculations

Calculations are an integral part of pharmacy practice. Whether it's figuring out prices or determining a patient-specific dose, pharmacists and technicians use arithmetic and simple algebra many times every day.

The good news is that virtually every common problem in pharmacy can be solved by using the mathematical technique known as *ratio and proportion*. By thinking through what you know and what you're trying to figure out, ratio and proportion will enable you to determine the answer easily by simply cross multiplying and then dividing. Let's look at this technique and then consider some practical applications.

If you are having trouble with these calculations, obtain a book that has a more in-depth presentation of calculations. You may find that another book in the APhA Pharmacy Technician Training Series, *Complete Math Review for the Pharmacy Technician* by William A. Hopkins, Jr., now in its second edition, will provide you with a more extensive presentation of all that is involved in pharmaceutical calculations.

Ratio and Proportion

When using the ratio and proportion method, set up two common fractions, one showing what you know and one containing the value that you're trying to calculate. For instance, suppose you want to know how many milligrams are in 0.5 g. As shown in Table 2-1, you can see that 1 g is equivalent to 1000 mg. Keep the units the same above each line and below each line. Thus, the following ratios can be set up:

$$\frac{1000\ mg}{1\ g} = \frac{?}{0.5\ g}$$

This can be read as, "1000 mg is to 1 g as the unknown quantity is to 0.5 g."

By cross multiplying the top of each fraction (the *numerators*) by the bottom of the other fraction (the *denominators*), you get the following equation:

$$\frac{1000\ mg}{1\ g} \diagdown\kern-1.2em\diagup \frac{?}{0.5\ g}$$

$$?\times 1\ g = 1000\ mg \times 0.5\ g$$

Now move all the numbers to the right side of the equation and leave only the ? on the left. You can do this by dividing both sides by 1 g and canceling common units. The calculations on the right then provide your answer:

$$? = \frac{1000\ mg \times 0.5\ g}{1\ g}$$

$$? = 1000\ mg \times 0.5$$

$$? = 500\ mg$$

You can quickly solve problems by converting most calculations into this format. Just remember—always set up two proportions, one showing the information you're given or what you know and the other putting the question mark in the appropriate place, depending on the information you're looking for.

> *The good news is that virtually every common problem in pharmacy can be solved by using the mathematical technique known as ratio and proportion.*

Metric Measures: Prefixes and Units of Weight, Length, and Volume

PREFIXES

kilo = 1000 times (abbreviated k)

deci = $\frac{1}{10}$ times (0.1; abbreviated d)

centi = $\frac{1}{100}$ times (0.01; abbreviated c)

milli = $\frac{1}{1000}$ times (0.001; abbreviated m)

micro = $\frac{1}{1,000,000}$ times (0.000001; abbreviated mc or μ)

WEIGHT (ALSO REFERRED TO AS MASS)

Basic unit: gram (g)

Units commonly encountered:

milligrams (mg), as in 1 g = 1000 mg

micrograms (mcg or μg), as in 1 mcg = 0.001 mg

kilogram (kg), as in 1 kg = 1000 g

LENGTH

Basic unit: meter (m)

Units commonly encountered:

centimeters (cm), as in 100 cm = 1 m

millimeters (mm), as in 1 cm = 10 mm = 0.01 m

VOLUME

Basic unit: liter (L)

Units commonly encountered:

milliliter (mL), as in 1 L = 1000 mL

deciliter (dL), as in 100 mL = 1 dL = 0.1 L

Units of Measure and Common Equivalents

A common type of calculation in pharmacy is converting between *metric measurements* (Table 2-1) and common equivalents, such as pounds, inches, or quarts, that you typically encounter in the United States. The common system is also called the *avoirdupois* (pronounced AV-WA-DU-PWA) *system*, and it uses the units shown in Table 2-2.

Pharmacy uses a third set of measures, the *apothecary system*, which you may see occasionally, even though it is now largely unused (Table 2-3). In the apothecary system, remember that the grains are the same as grains in the avoirdupois system, but the ounces and pounds are different. While you will occasionally see drug doses expressed in grains and scruples, the PTCB examination does not include any items that test your knowledge of this antiquated system. The three drugs for which the apothecary system continues to be used most often are aspirin (a 325-mg aspirin tablet contains 5 grains of this drug), thyroid products, and phenobarbital.

Avoirdupois Units of Weight, Length, and Volume

WEIGHT	LENGTH	VOLUME
Basic unit: ounce (oz)	Basic unit: inch (in)	Basic unit: ounce
Units commonly encountered:	*Units commonly encountered:*	*Units commonly encountered:*
1 oz = 437.5 grains (gr)	12 in = 1 foot (ft)	8 oz = 1 cup
1 pound (lb) = 16 oz = 7000 gr	3 ft = 1 yard (yd)	2 cups = 1 pint (pt)
		2 pt = 1 quart (qt)
		4 qt = 1 gallon (gal)

TABLE 2-3

Apothecary Units of Weight and Volume[a]

WEIGHT

Basic unit: grain (gr)

Units commonly encountered:

    20 gr = 1 scruple (℈)

    3 scruples = 1 dram (ℨ)

    8 drams = 1 oz (℥)

    12 oz = 1 pound (lb)

VOLUME

Basic unit: minim (♏)

Units commonly encountered:

    60 minims = 1 fluid dram

    8 fluid drams = 1 fluid oz

    16 fluid ounces = 1 pt

    2 pt = 1 qt

    4 qt = 1 gal

[a] *The PTCB examination does not test on knowledge of this system.*

Table 2-4 shows the mathematical relationships among the metric, apothecary, and avoirdupois systems.

These various units and systems give us a good chance to try using ratio and proportion to solve simple problems. Here are examples of questions you may encounter and problems you can use to test yourself (answers to those problems not solved for you are shown at the end of this chapter).

1. How many inches are in 4 feet?

$$\frac{12 \text{ in}}{1 \text{ ft}} = \frac{?}{4 \text{ ft}}$$

$? \times 1 \text{ ft} = 12 \text{ in} \times 4 \text{ ft}$

$$? = \frac{12 \text{ in} \times 4 \text{ ft}}{1 \text{ ft}}$$

$? = 12 \text{ in} \times 4$

$? = 48 \text{ in}$

2. How many milligrams are in 4 grams?

$$\frac{1000 \text{ mg}}{1 \text{ g}} = \frac{?}{4 \text{ g}}$$

$? \times 1 \text{ g} = 1000 \text{ mg} \times 4 \text{ g}$

$$? = \frac{1000 \text{ mg} \times 4 \text{ g}}{1 \text{ g}}$$

$? = 1000 \text{ mg} \times 4$

$? = 4000 \text{ mg}$

3. How many milligrams are in 5 grains?

$$\frac{65 \text{ mg}}{1 \text{ gr}} = \frac{?}{5 \text{ gr}}$$

$? \times 1 \text{ gr} = 65 \text{ mg} \times 5 \text{ gr}$

$$? = \frac{65 \text{ mg} \times 5 \text{ gr}}{1 \text{ gr}}$$

$? = 65 \text{ mg} \times 5$

$? = 325 \text{ mg}$

Note: As mentioned earlier in this chapter, a 5-gr aspirin tablet therefore contains 325 mg. This is also the weight of a regular-dose acetaminophen (Tylenol) tablet or capsule.

4. How many kilograms does a 154-pound person weigh?

$$\frac{1 \text{ kg}}{2.2 \text{ lb}} = \frac{?}{154 \text{ lb}}$$

$? \times 2.2 \text{ lb} = 1 \text{ kg} \times 154 \text{ lb}$

$$? = \frac{1 \text{ kg} \times 154 \text{ lb}}{2.2 \text{ lb}}$$

$$? = \frac{154 \text{ kg}}{2.2}$$

$? = 70 \text{ kg}$

Did you know? Most pharmacokinetic calculations—those used by pharmacists to calculate drug dosages—are based on a 70-kg person. The equations are adjusted for the patient's actual body mass as part of the calculation.

5. How many milliliters are in 1 quart?

   Tip: First convert the quart unit to ounces, then solve for milliliters!

   1 qt = 2 pt = 32 oz

   $$\frac{30\ mL}{1\ oz} = \frac{?}{32\ oz}$$

   ? × 1 oz = 30 mL × 32 oz

   $$? = \frac{30\ mL \times 32\ oz}{1\ oz}$$

   ? = 30 mL × 32

   ? = 960 mL

   Now you complete some problems!

6. How many grams are in 3 kilograms?

   $$\frac{1000\ g}{1\ kg} = \frac{?}{3\ kg}$$

7. How many milliliters are in 5 dL?

   $$\frac{100\ mL}{1\ dL} = \frac{?}{5\ dL}$$

8. How many inches are in 5 meters?

   $$\frac{39.4\ in}{1\ m} = \frac{?}{5\ m}$$

9. If a patient weighs 22.4 kilograms, how many pounds is that?

   $$\frac{1\ kg}{2.2\ lb} = \frac{22.4\ kg}{?}$$

   A new way to diet: Just give your weight in kilograms!

10. How many avoirdupois ounces are in 1 kg?

    Tip: Use the 1 oz (avoirdupois) = 28.4 g conversion,
    but convert the grams to kilograms by dividing it by 1000 ($\frac{28.4}{1000} = 0.0284\ kg$).

    $$\frac{1\ oz}{0.0284\ kg} = \frac{?}{1\ kg}$$

    ? × 0.0284 kg = 1 oz × 1 kg

    $$? = \frac{1\ oz \times 1\ kg}{0.0284\ kg}$$

    $$? = \frac{1}{0.0284\ oz}$$

11. How many centimeters are in 6 inches?

12. How many milliliters are in 15 liters?

13. If an extra-strength tablet of Tylenol contains 500 mg of acetaminophen,
    how many grams are in 100 tablets? How many grams are in 1 tablet?

    Hint: For the first part of this problem, the proportion would be : $\frac{500\ mg}{1\ tablet} = \frac{?}{100\ tablets}$
    After you get an answer in milligrams, convert it to grams.

TABLE 2-4

Metric, Apothecary,ᵃ and Avoirdupois Conversions

LENGTH

1 m = 39.4 in

1 in = 2.54 cm

VOLUME

1 fluid oz (f℥) = 30 mL

1 pt = 473 mL

1 gal = 3,785 mL

WEIGHT

1 kg = 2.2 lb avoirdupois

1 lb avoirdupois = 454 g

1 oz avoirdupois (℥) = 28.4 g

1 oz apothecary = 31 g

1 g = 15.4 grains (gr)

1 gr = 65 mg

ᵃ The PTCB examination does not test on knowledge of the apothecary system or conversions to and from it.

14. If a solution has 10 mg of drug per milliliter, how much drug is in 10 mL?

Hint: $\dfrac{10\ mg}{1\ mL} = \dfrac{?}{10\ mL}$

Percentage Calculations

While most medications are commercially available in ready-to-dispense form, pharmacists and pharmacy technicians sometimes make prescriptions from other ingredients through a process called compounding. This process will be described in more detail in Chapters 9 and 10.

Percentage calculations come into play during compounding when one substance (usually the drug) is dissolved or incorporated into a larger amount of a second substance. This is most often a solution in which a drug powder is dissolved in water or some other vehicle. The percentage then refers to the amount of drug (the *solute*) that is dispersed in the vehicle (the *solvent*). An example would be a solution of salt, or sodium chloride, dissolved in water.

Many of these products are prepared for injection into the veins, and many contain very powerful drugs. Because there is little room for error in these or any other pharmaceutical calculations, you need to be completely certain of the accuracy of your work; double or triple check your calculations or ask someone else to confirm them.

Fortunately, percentage calculations can be solved using the same ratio and proportion technique presented in Units of Measure and Common Equivalents. All you have to remember is what "percentage" means: the amount of solute in grams or milliliters contained in 100 mL or 100 g of the final solution. For instance, if 5 g of dextrose (the chemical name for table sugar) is dissolved in water such that 100 mL of total solution is prepared, the result is a 5% solution of dextrose in water. Because this type of solution involves a certain weight of drug in a total volume of solution, it is sometimes called a *weight-to-volume* solution, and you will sometimes see the concentration expressed as 5% w/v to denote this relationship. But because this is the most common kind of solution, it is often understood that the percentage is w/v if nothing indicates otherwise.

An example involving two liquids would be alcohol dissolved in water. A 70% ethanol solution in water is made up of 70 mL of ethanol (the kind of alcohol found in beer, wine, and liquor) mixed with enough water to make 100 mL of solution. These types of solutions are sometimes called *volume-in-volume* solutions, and the percentage is then written as 70% v/v.

When a drug is incorporated into another solid or semisolid product, such as a cream or ointment, the product is expressed as a *weight-in-weight* percentage. For example, 2 g of lidocaine mixed with enough of a compounding base to make 100 g of ointment would be a 2% w/w lidocaine ointment.

Let's try a few problems using percentage calculations.

15. How many grams of dextrose are in 50 mL of a 5% *w/v* solution?

First, set up two common fractions that express the proportional relationships:

$$\frac{5\ g}{100\ mL} = \frac{?}{50\ mL}$$

$$? \times 100\ mL = 5\ g \times 50\ mL$$

$$? = \frac{5\ g \times 50\ mL}{100\ mL}$$

$$? = \frac{5\ g \times 50}{100}$$

$$? = 2.5\ g$$

16. How many liters of a 5% dextrose solution contain 100 g of dextrose?

$$\frac{5 \text{ g}}{100 \text{ mL}} = \frac{100 \text{ g}}{?}$$

$? \times 5 \text{ g} = 100 \text{ mL} \times 100 \text{ g}$

$$? = \frac{100 \text{ mL} \times 100 \text{ g}}{5 \text{ g}}$$

$$? = \frac{100 \text{ mL} \times 100}{5}$$

$? = 2000 \text{ mL}$

Now, convert 2000 mL to liters:

$$\frac{1000 \text{ mL}}{1 \text{ L}} = \frac{2000 \text{ mL}}{?}$$

$? \times 1000 \text{ mL} = 1 \text{ L} \times 2000 \text{ mL}$

$$? = \frac{1 \text{ L} \times 2000 \text{ mL}}{1000 \text{ mL}}$$

$$? = \frac{1 \text{ L} \times 2000}{1000}$$

$? = 2 \text{ L}$

17. How many grams of lidocaine are in 75 g of a 2% *w/w* ointment?

$$\frac{2 \text{ g of lidocaine}}{100 \text{ g of ointment}} = \frac{?}{75 \text{ g of ointment}}$$

$? \times 100 \text{ g of ointment} = 2 \text{ g of lidocaine} \times 75 \text{ g of ointment}$

$$? = 2 \text{ g of lidocaine} \times \frac{75 \text{ g of ointment}}{100 \text{ g of ointment}}$$

$$? = 2 \text{ g of lidocaine} \times \frac{75}{100}$$

$? = 1.5 \text{ g of lidocaine}$

18. How many milliliters of ethanol are in 35 mL of a 70% *v/v* ethanol solution?

$$\frac{70 \text{ mL of ethanol}}{100 \text{ mL of solution}} = \frac{?}{35 \text{ mL of solution}}$$

$? \times 100 \text{ mL of solution} = 70 \text{ mL of ethanol} \times 35 \text{ mL of solution}$

$$? = 70 \text{ mL of ethanol} \times \frac{35 \text{ mL of solution}}{100 \text{ mL of solution}}$$

$$? = \frac{70 \text{ mL of ethanol} \times 35}{100}$$

$? = 24.5 \text{ mL of ethanol}$

19. **How many grams of a 1% hydrocortisone cream contain 0.5 g of hydrocortisone?**

$$\frac{1 \text{ g of hydrocortisone}}{100 \text{ g of cream}} = \frac{0.5 \text{ g of hydrocortisone}}{?}$$

$? \times 1 \text{ g of hydrocortisone} = 100 \text{ g of cream} \times 0.5 \text{ g of hydrocortisone}$

$? = 100 \text{ g of cream} \times \dfrac{0.5 \text{ g of hydrocortisone}}{1 \text{ g of hydrocortisone}}$

$? = 100 \text{ g of cream} \times \dfrac{0.5}{1}$

$? = 50 \text{ g of cream}$

20. **How much sodium chloride is in 200 mL of a 0.9% solution?**

$$\frac{0.9 \text{ g}}{100 \text{ mL}} = \frac{?}{200 \text{ mL}}$$

$? \times 100 \text{ mL} = 0.9 \text{ g} \times 200 \text{ mL}$

$? = 0.9 \text{ g} \times \dfrac{200 \text{ mL}}{100 \text{ mL}}$

$? = 0.9 \text{ g} \times \dfrac{200}{100}$

$? = 1.8 \text{ g}$

21. **How much of a 70% *v/v* ethanol solution would contain 140 mL of ethanol?**

$$\frac{70 \text{ mL ethanol}}{100 \text{ mL solution}} = \frac{140 \text{ mL ethanol}}{?}$$

$? \times 70 \text{ mL ethanol} = 100 \text{ mL solution} \times 140 \text{ mL ethanol}$

$? = 100 \text{ mL solution} \times \dfrac{140 \text{ mL ethanol}}{70 \text{ mL ethanol}}$

$? = 100 \text{ mL solution} \times \dfrac{140}{70}$

$? = 200 \text{ mL solution}$

Now try some on your own.

22. **How many grams of dextrose would be needed to make 300 mL of a 5% dextrose solution?**

$$\frac{5 \text{ g}}{100 \text{ mL}} = \frac{?}{300 \text{ mL}}$$

23. **How many milliliters of ethanol are in 50 mL of a 50% *v/v* solution?**

24. **To prepare 150 g of a 2% *w/w* lidocaine ointment, how many grams of lidocaine would you need?**

Similar to
percentage
calculations,
ratio strength
problems can be
weight-in-volume,
volume-in-volume,
or weight-in-weight,
depending on
whether the
preparation
involves liquids
or solids.

Ratio Strengths

Ratio strengths are another type of pharmaceutical calculation that are quite similar to percentage concentration problems. The amount of drug in a preparation is expressed as a ratio strength (for example, a 1:10 strength).

Similar to percentage calculations, ratio strength problems can be weight-in-volume, volume-in-volume, or weight-in-weight, depending on whether the preparation involves liquids or solids. As above, this calculation most often involves a solution in which a drug powder is dissolved in water or some other vehicle. But it could be a liquid dissolved in a liquid, as with alcohol in water, or a mixture of two solids, as with a drug in a cream or ointment. The percentage refers to the amount of drug (the solute) that is dispersed in the vehicle (the solvent).

With ratio strengths, you always assume that the solute is 1 part. Then you calculate how many parts of the final preparation contain that 1 part. For instance, in a 1:10 solution of sodium chloride, there is 1 part of sodium chloride in 10 parts of solution. This is basically the opposite of a percentage calculation where you are calculating the amount of solute present in 100 g or 100 mL of final product.

Here are some examples of ratio strength problems.

25. **What is the ratio strength (*w/v*) of a solution with 2 g of drug in 50 mL of solution?**
First, set up two common fractions that express the proportional relationships:

$$\frac{1\ g}{?} = \frac{2\ g}{50\ mL}$$

$$? \times 2\ g = 1\ g \times 50\ mL$$

$$? = 1\ g \times \frac{50\ mL}{2\ g}$$

$$? = 1 \times \frac{50\ mL}{2}$$

$$? = 25\ mL$$

Therefore, the ratio strength is expressed as 1:25.

26. **How many liters of a 1:20 dextrose solution contain 100 g of dextrose?**

$$\frac{100\ g}{?} = \frac{1\ g}{20\ mL}$$

$$? \times 1\ g = 100\ g \times 20\ mL$$

$$? = 100\ g \times \frac{20\ mL}{1\ g}$$

$$? = 100 \times \frac{20\ mL}{1}$$

$$? = 2000\ mL$$

$$\frac{1000\ mL}{1\ L} = \frac{2000\ mL}{?}$$

$$? \times 1000\ mL = 1\ L \times 2000\ mL$$

$$? = 1\ L \times \frac{2000\ mL}{1000\ mL}$$

$$? = 1\ L \times \frac{2000}{1000}$$

$$? = 2\ L$$

27. **How many grams of lidocaine are in 75 g of a 1:50 *w/w* ointment?**

$$\frac{1 \text{ g of lidocaine}}{50 \text{ g of ointment}} = \frac{?}{75 \text{ g of ointment}}$$

$? \times 50 \text{ g of ointment} = 1 \text{ g of lidocaine} \times 75 \text{ g of ointment}$

$? = 1 \text{ g of lidocaine} \times \dfrac{75 \text{ g of ointment}}{50 \text{ g of ointment}}$

$? = 1 \text{g of lidocaine} \times \dfrac{75}{50}$

$? = 1.5 \text{ g of lidocaine}$

28. **How many milliliters of ethanol are in 35 mL of a 1:2 *v/v* ethanol solution?**

$$\frac{1 \text{ mL of ethanol}}{2 \text{ mL of solution}} = \frac{?}{35 \text{ mL of solution}}$$

$? \times 2 \text{ mL of solution} = 1 \text{ mL of ethanol} \times 35 \text{ mL of solution}$

$? = 1 \text{ mL of ethanol} \times \dfrac{35 \text{ mL of solution}}{2 \text{ mL of solution}}$

$? = 100 \text{ mL of ethanol} \times \dfrac{35}{2}$

$? = 17.5 \text{ mL of ethanol}$

29. **How many grams of a 1:100 hydrocortisone cream contain 0.5 g of hydrocortisone?**

$$\frac{1 \text{ g of hydrocortisone}}{100 \text{ g of cream}} = \frac{0.5 \text{ g of hydrocortisone}}{?}$$

$? \times 1 \text{ g of hydrocortisone} = 100 \text{ g of cream} \times 0.5 \text{ g of hydrocortisone}$

$? = 100 \text{ g of cream} \times \dfrac{0.5 \text{ g of hydrocortisone}}{1 \text{ g of hydrocortisone}}$

$? = 100 \text{ g of cream} \times \dfrac{0.5}{1}$

$? = 50 \text{ g of cream}$

30. **How much sodium chloride is in 200 mL of a 1:111 solution?**

$$\frac{1 \text{ g}}{111 \text{ mL}} = \frac{?}{200 \text{ mL}}$$

$? \times 111 \text{ mL} = 1 \text{ g} \times 200 \text{ mL}$

$? = 1 \text{ g} \times \dfrac{200 \text{ mL}}{111 \text{ mL}}$

$? = 1 \text{ g} \times \dfrac{200}{111}$

$? = 1.8 \text{ g}$

31. How much of a 1:1.43 *v/v* ethanol solution would contain 140 mL of ethanol?

$$\frac{1 \text{ mL ethanol}}{1.43 \text{ mL solution}} = \frac{140 \text{ mL ethanol}}{?}$$

$$? \times 1 \text{ mL ethanol} = 1.43 \text{ mL solution} \times 140 \text{ mL ethanol}$$

$$? = 1.43 \text{ mL solution} \times \frac{140 \text{ mL ethanol}}{1 \text{ mL ethanol}}$$

$$? = 1.43 \text{ mL solution} \times \frac{140}{1}$$

$$? = 200 \text{ mL solution}$$

Here are some problems for you to try.

32. How many grams of dexamethasone are in 75 g of a 1:100 cream?

33. How many liters of a 1:2 alcohol solution contain 4 L of alcohol?

34. How many grams of dextrose are in 300 mL of a 1:20 solution?

Temperature Conversion

Most temperature measurements in medicine are taken using the Centigrade or Celsius system, while Americans are more familiar with Fahrenheit temperatures. Occasionally, pharmacy technicians are called on to convert between the two systems. The Celsius scale is based on the freezing and boiling points of water, which are denoted as 0°C and 100°C. These two points are equivalent to 32°F and 212°F. Thus, to convert between the two systems, this equation is used:

$$9(°C) = 5(°F) - 160$$

Let's use this equation to solve some problems.

35. Convert 39°F to °C.

$$9(°C) = 5(°F) - 160$$
$$9(°C) = 5(39) - 160$$
$$9(°C) = 195 - 160$$
$$9(°C) = 35$$
$$°C = \frac{35}{9}$$
$$°C = 3.9$$

36. Convert 80°C to °F.

$$9(°C) = 5(°F) - 160$$
$$9(80°) = 5(°F) - 160$$
$$5(°F) = 720 + 160$$
$$5(°F) = 880$$
$$°F = \frac{880}{5}$$
$$°F = 176$$

Now try some problems on your own.

37. Convert 98.6°F (normal body temperature) to °C.

38. Convert 20°C to °F.

Household Equivalents

In the community and ambulatory pharmacy settings, patients need to use common household measures to administer liquid medications. Table 2-5 provides conversions between metric quantities and household measurements. Let's use the conversions to calculate drug dosages.

TABLE 2-5

Common Household Equivalents of Metric Liquid Measures

METRIC MEASURE (mL)	HOUSEHOLD EQUIVALENT
5	1 teaspoonful (tsp)
15	1 tablespoonful (Tbs) or 3 tsp
30 (equal to 1 fluid oz)	2 Tbs

39. How much drug is in 2 tsp of a $\dfrac{10 \text{ mg}}{5 \text{ mL}}$ solution?

First, convert the common household measure to the metric system using ratio and proportion.

$$\frac{1 \text{ tsp}}{5 \text{ mL}} = \frac{2 \text{ tsp}}{?}$$

$$? \times 1 \text{ tsp} = 5 \text{ mL} \times 2 \text{ tsp}$$

$$? = 5 \text{ mL} \times \frac{2 \text{ tsp}}{1 \text{ tsp}}$$

$$? = 5 \text{ mL} \times \frac{2}{1}$$

$$? = 10 \text{ mL}$$

Then, calculate the amount of drug in the 10 mL using ratio and proportion.

$$\frac{10 \text{ mg}}{5 \text{ mL}} = \frac{?}{10 \text{ mL}}$$

$$? \times 5 \text{ mL} = 10 \text{ mg} \times 10 \text{ mL}$$

$$? = 10 \text{ mg} \times \frac{10 \text{ mL}}{5 \text{ mL}}$$

$$? = 10 \text{ mg} \times \frac{10}{5}$$

$$? = 20 \text{ mg}$$

40. How many teaspoonfuls are in a 1-pt bottle of medication?

Since 1 pint contains 473 mL and 1 tsp is 5 mL, the following ratio and proportion can be set up:

$$\frac{1 \text{ tsp}}{5 \text{ mL}} = \frac{?}{473 \text{ mL}}$$

$$? \times 5 \text{ mL} = 1 \text{ tsp} \times 473 \text{ mL}$$

$$? = 1 \text{ tsp} \times \frac{473 \text{ mL}}{5 \text{ mL}}$$

$$? = 1 \text{ tsp} \times \frac{473}{5}$$

$$? = 94.6 \text{ tsp (meaning that 94 full teaspoonfuls can be obtained from a 1-pt bottle)}$$

Now try some calculations on your own.

41. How many 1-Tbs (tablespoonful) doses can be obtained from a 90-mL bottle of medicine?

42. If an antibiotic suspension has $\frac{150 \text{ mg}}{5 \text{ mL}}$, how much drug is in 1 tablespoonful?

Pharmaceutical Abbreviations

When doctors write prescriptions, they use abbreviations for Latin terms that tell pharmacists how patients are to take the medications. For instance, instead of writing "two times a day," they just write "bid," which is an abbreviation for two times a day in Latin.

Table 2-6 lists the most commonly used abbreviations, and you will need to memorize them. To help you learn these abbreviations, notice certain commonalities:

a can be an abbreviation for *ante*, meaning *before*, or *aura*, meaning *ear*.

d can mean *die*, for *day*, or *dextro*, meaning *right*.

h stands for *hora* or hour.

b, *t*, and *q* usually refer to how many times a day to give a medicine, standing for two times, three times, and four times daily, respectively.

q stands for *quaque*, meaning *every*.

o stands for *oculo*, for eye.

Examples:

ac	=	before meals
ad	=	right ear
qd	=	every day
q 4 h	=	every 4 hours
bid	=	two times a day
tid	=	three times a day
qid	=	four times a day
qd	=	every day
q 8 h	=	every 8 hours
od	=	right eye
os	=	left eye

TABLE 2-6

Common Pharmaceutical Abbreviations Used on Prescriptions

LATIN-BASED ABBREVIATIONS

a	before
ac	before meals
ad	right ear
as	left ear
au	both ears or each ear
bid	two times a day
c	with
dtd	dispense such doses
gtt, gtts	drop or drops
h, hr	hour
hs	at bedtime (at the hour of sleep)
non rep	do not repeat, no refills
p	after
po	by mouth
prn	as needed
q	every
qd	every day
q am	every morning
q pm	every evening
q hs	every bedtime
qod	every other day (every second day)

q 4 h	every 4 hours (or 3, 6, 8, 12, 24, or other intervals)
qid	four times a day
tid	three times a day
os	left eye
od	right eye
ou	both eyes or each eye
ut dict, ud	as directed
stat	at once, now

OTHER COMMON ABBREVIATIONS

APAP	acetaminophen
ASA	aspirin
DAW	dispense as written
IM	intramuscular
IV	intravenous
MOM	milk of magnesia
NSAID	nonsteroidal anti-inflammatory drug
OTC	over-the-counter (as in nonprescription)
PCN	penicillin
SC	subcutaneous
TCN	tetracycline

Medical Terminology

While the words used to describe parts of the body, medical procedures, and diseases can certainly be formidable, many of them can be broken down to common prefixes, roots, and suffixes that help you deduce their meaning. A complete discussion of medical terminology cannot be offered in this brief textbook, but this section will give you some tools to use in beginning to understand complex medical terminology. According to *Stedman's Medical Dictionary*, about 400 such word parts make up 90% to 95% of all medical terminology. By learning these word parts, you can decipher most medical terms, even if you have never encountered them before.

The most common of these 400 word parts are shown in Table 2-7 with explanatory examples. The entries under "prefixes and combining forms" are used at the beginning of words, in the middle of terms, or with root words, as follows:

an- (without) + hedonia (pleasure) = anhedonia (without pleasure)

poly- (many) + dactyl (fingers or toes) = polydactyly (having more than five fingers or toes)

Similarly, suffixes can be added to prefixes, combining forms, or root words to form medical terms, as follows:

splen- (referring to the spleen) + -ectomy (removal) = splenectomy (removal of the spleen)

laryng- (referring to the larynx) + -itis (inflammation) = laryngitis (loss of voice caused by inflammation of the larynx, or voice box)

TABLE 2-7

Common Medical Prefixes and Suffixes, Their Meanings, and Examples

ELEMENT	MEANING	EXAMPLE	ELEMENT	MEANING	EXAMPLE
Prefixes and Combining Forms			enter-, entero-	intestines	gastroenterology
a-, an-	without	aplastic, anhedonia	erythro-	red	erythrocyte (red blood cell)
arteri-, arterio-	artery	arteriosclerosis			
arthro-	bone joint	arthroscope	eu-	good, well	eugenics, eutectic
auto-	self	autoimmune	ex-	out, away from	exhalation
bacteri-, bacterio-	bacteria	bacteriostatic	extra-	without, outside of	extrachromosomal
bi-	twice, double	bisexual, binocular	ferri-, ferro-	iron	ferric sulfate, ferrous citrate
bronch-, bronchi-	bronchus	bronchitis			
carcin-, carcino-	cancer	carcinogenic	gloss-	tongue	glossitis
cardi, cardio-	heart	cardiology	gyn-, gyne-, gyneco-, gyno-	woman	gynecology
chlor-, chloro-	chlorine	hydrochloric acid			
chol-	bile	cholestasis	hem-, hema-, hemat-, hemato-	blood	hematology, hemoglobin
chondro-	cartilage	chondrocyte			
cis-	on the same side as (chemistry)	cis-retinoic acid (see trans-)	hist-, histio-	tissue	histology
			hydr-, hydro-	water, hydrogen	hydrolysis
co-, col-, com-, con-, cor-	together with	cofactor	hyper-	excessive, above normal	hyperactive
crani-, cranio-	cranium (head, skull)	craniotomy	hypo-	beneath, less than normal	hypotonic
cry-	cold	cryogenic	hyster-	uterus	hysterectomy
cyst-	bladder	cystitis	ileo-	ileum (small intestine)	ileotomy
cyt-	cell	cytology			
dactyl-	fingers, toes	dactyledema	infra-	below	infrared
de-	away, cessation	decompose	inter-	among, between	intervascular (between blood and lymph vessels)
derm-	skin	dermatology			
dextr-	toward the right	dextroamphetamine			
duodeno-	duodenum (small intestine)	duodenal ulcer	intra-	within	intravenous (within veins)
			irid-	iris (of the eye)	iridology, iritis
dys-	bad, difficult	dysfunctional	kerat-, kerato-	cornea (of the eye)	keratectomy
ect-	outer, outside	ectoderm			
encephalo-	brain	encephalogram	kinesi-, kinesio-	movement	kinesiology
end-, endo-	within, inner	endoderm	lact-, lacto-	milk	lactose, lactase

TABLE 2-7 (continued)

Common Medical Prefixes and Suffixes, Their Meanings, and Examples

ELEMENT	MEANING	EXAMPLE
laryng-	larynx (in the throat)	laryngitis
latero-	to one side	lateral, lateroflexion
lepto-	frail, slender, thin	leptin
leuko-	white	leukocyte (white blood cell)
lip-, lipo-	fat, lipid	liposome
lymph-	lymph system, glands	lymphatic
lys-	breaking up, dissolution	lysis
macro-	large	macrocyte
mast-, masto-	breast	mastectomy
meg-, mega-, megalo-	large	megalocytes
melan-, melano-	black	melanoma
mening-, meningo-	meninges	meningitis
morph-, morpho-	form, shape, structure	morphology
myx-, myxo-	mucus	myxedema, myxoid
necr-, necro-	death	necrosis
nephr-, nephro-	kidney	nephritis, nephrology
neur-, neuri-, neuro-	nerve, nervous system	neurology
oculo-	eye	oculoscope
olig-, oligo-	few, little	oligospermia
onco-	tumor	oncology
onych-, onycho-	fingernail, toenail	onychectomy
oo-, oophor-, oophoro-	ovary, ovum	oophorectomy
ophthalm-, ophthalmo-	eyes	ophthalmology
orchi-, orchido-, orchio-	testis	orchidectomy
ossi-, osseo-, ost-, oste-, osteo-	bone	osteoporosis
ovari-, ovario-	ovary	ovariectomy
ovi-, ovo-	egg	oviduct
oxa-, oxo-	addition of oxygen	oxalic acid, oxalate
pan-, pant-, panto-	all, entire	pandemic (worldwide epidemic)

ELEMENT	MEANING	EXAMPLE
path-, patho-	disease	pathology
ped-, pedi-, pedo-	child or foot	pediatrics, pedograph
peri-	around	pericardium
pharmaco-	drugs, medicine	pharmacotherapy
pharyng-, pharyngo-	pharynx (of the throat)	pharyngotomy
phleb-, phlebo-	vein	phlebotomy
phos-, phot-, photo-	light	photophobic
phren-, phreni-	diaphragm	phrenoplegia
physi-, physio-	physical, natural	physiology
plasma-, plasmat-, plasmato-	plasma	plasmapheresis
pleur-, pleura-, pleuro-	rib, side, pleura	pleural, pleurisy
pneum-, pneuma-, pneumata-, pneumato-	air, gas, lungs, breathing	pneumonitis
poly-	multiple	polydactyly, polyuria
post-	after, behind	postpartum (after childbirth)
pre-	before	preprandial (before eating)
pro-	before, precursor of	prodrug
proct-, procto-	anus, rectum	proctologist
psych-, psyche-, psycho-	mind	psychopathology
pyel-, pyelo-	renal pelvis	pyelonephritis
pyreto-, pyro-	heat, fever	pyretics (drugs that relieve fever)
radio-	radiation, x-rays	radiology
re-, retro-	again, backward	reconstructive, retro-grade
rhin-, rhino-	nose	rhinitis
schiz-, schizo-	split, cleft, division	schizophrenia
scler-, sclero-	hardness, the sclera	scleroderma
semi-	one half, partly	semicomatose
sigmoid-, sigmoido-	sigmoid colon (large intestine)	sigmoidoscopy
somat-, somato-, somatico-	the body	somatotropic

TABLE 2-7 (continued)

Common Medical Prefixes and Suffixes, Their Meanings, and Examples

ELEMENT	MEANING	EXAMPLE	ELEMENT	MEANING	EXAMPLE
spermato-, spermo-, sperma-	semen, sperm	spermatozoa	**Suffixes**		
			-ase	an enzyme	sucrase
splen-, spleno-	spleen	splenectomy	-ate	a salt or ester of an acid	sulfate
staphyl-, staphylo-	staphylococci	staphylococcal			
steno-	narrowness, constriction	stenosis	-cidal, -cide	killing, destroying	bactericidal
			-cyte	cell	macrocyte
stom-, stoma-, stomat-, stomato-	mouth	stomatitis	-ectomy	excision, removal	splenectomy
			-gram	recording	electrocardiogram
sub-	beneath, less than normal	subdural	-graph	recording instrument	polygraph
super-	in excess, above, superior	supersaturate, superovulation	-ia, -iasis	condition	trichomoniasis
			-ic	pertaining to	physiologic
therm-, thermo-	heat	thermometer	-ism	condition, disease	trophism
thorac-, thoracico-	chest, thorax	thoracotomy	-itis	inflammation	nephritis
thromb-, thrombo-	blood clot	thrombosis	-lepsis, -lepsy	seizure	epilepsy
thyr-, thyro-	thyroid gland	thyrotoxicosis	-ology	study of	biology, nephrology
toco-	childbirth	tocolytic	-megaly	large	acromegaly
tox-, toxico-, toxo-	toxin, poison	toxicology	-oid	resemblance to	lymphoid
trache-, tracheo-	trachea	tracheotomy	-oma, -omata	tumor, neoplasm	keratoma
trans-	across (chemical designation)	trans-retinoic acid (see cis-)	-one	chemical ketone group	acetone
trich-, trichi-, trichia-, tricho-	hair, hairlike structure	trichitis	-otomy	incision, cutting into	lobotomy
tropho-	food, nutrition	trophoblast, trophoderm	-pathy	disease	cardiopathy
			-penia	deficiency	leukopenia
uri-, uric-, urico-	uric acid	uricosuric	-phage, -phagia	eating	polyphagia
vas-	duct, blood vessel	vas deferens	-phobe, phobic	afraid of	claustrophobic
vasculo-, vaso-	blood vessel	vasculogenesis	-plegia	paralysis	paraplegia
vesic-, vesico-	vesica, vesicle	vesiculitis	-poiesis	production	hematopoiesis
zo-, zoo-	animal, animal life	zoonoses	-rrhagia, -rrhage	discharge	hemorrhage
zy-	fertilization	zygote, zygospore	-rrhea	flowing	rhinorrhea, diarrhea
zym-, zymo-	enzymes	zymology, zymogen	-scope	instrument for viewing	microscope
			-scopy	use of instrument for viewing	microscopy
			-stat	agent to prevent change	bacteriostat
			-trophic	food, nutrition	lymphotrophic
			-uria	urine	glycosuria

Now, using the information in Table 2-7, try to decipher the meaning of the following medical terms:

- photophobic
- stomatitis
- nephrectomy
- thoracotomy
- gastroscopy

Conclusion

While much of the information in this chapter requires memorization, it will serve you well as you begin to process prescriptions in the pharmacy. Through a minimal amount of memorization and a large measure of understanding the way calculations are performed, conversions are made, and words are formed, you will feel quite confident in your everyday duties and your interactions with pharmacists and other health care professionals.

In the next chapter, we consider the laws and regulations that govern the practice of pharmacy. Just as you need to know your own personal limits, you must know what controls the state and federal governments have placed on the practice of pharmacy.

For More Information

If you are preparing for the Pharmacy Technician Certification Examination and feel that you need more information about the topics discussed in this chapter, consider studying these sources of additional information:

- Hopkins WA Jr. *Complete Math Review for the Pharmacy Technician*, 2nd ed. Washington, D.C.: American Pharmacists Association; 2005.
- Snipe K. Prescription requirements and preparation. In: *The Pharmacy Technician Skills-Building Manual*. Washington, D.C.: American Pharmacists Association; 2007:43-62.

Reference

Stedman TL. *Stedman's Medical Dictionary*. 27th ed. Baltimore, MD: Lippincott Williams & Wilkins; 2000.

Answers to Unsolved Problems in This Chapter

6. 3,000
7. 500
8. 197
9. 49.28
10. 35.21
11. 15.24
12. 15,000
13. 50 (100 tablets); 0.5 (1 tablet)
14. 100
22. 15
23. 25
24. 3
32. 0.75
33. 8
34. 15
37. 37
38. 68
41. 6
42. 450

CHAPTER THREE

Pharmacy Governance

This chapter focuses on the Food and Drug Administration (FDA), the Centers for Medicare & Medicaid Services (CMS), the Drug Enforcement Administration (DEA), and state boards of pharmacy. It describes the drug-approval process and introduces FDA regulatory actions such as drug recalls. Then it covers DEA regulation of controlled substances in detail. Although state-specific board of pharmacy regulations cannot be covered, the chapter emphasizes the important roles that these agencies play in the daily operation and regulation of pharmacies.

Introduction

Because medications have such powerful effects on the human body and are such specialized entities, they are subject to many governmental rules and regulations at both the federal and state levels. Pharmacies, especially those in hospitals and those that serve nursing homes but also community pharmacies, are subject to additional governmental regulations tied to the ways those facilities are paid for pharmaceuticals and medication therapy management services with federal monies. In addition, the pharmacy profession regulates itself through voluntary programs involving accreditation of training programs and certification of individuals. In this chapter, these governmental and voluntary programs are described as they apply to you, the pharmacy technician.

Food and Drug Administration

The FDA is the part of the federal government that controls which medications can be legally sold in the United States. Its decisions have profound effects on medical care. The agency also oversees medical devices (including pumps used to infuse drugs), dietary supplements (herbal and alternative medicines), cosmetics and other beauty aids, and foods.

History

FDA was created through the passage of the Federal Food and Drug Act in 1906. In addition to oversight of foods, FDA initially had the authority to pursue manufacturers of pharmaceutical products that were *misbranded* (not truthful in labeling or promotions) or *adulterated* (not accurate as to contents or contaminated with other substances, microorganisms, trash, rodent excrement or matter, or other types of foreign matter).

In 1937, a terrible tragedy struck the country when a toxic preparation of Elixir Sulfanilamide caused 73 deaths. This tragedy resulted in passage of the Food, Drug, and Cosmetic Act of 1938, which expanded FDA's oversight to include approval of new drug products, medical devices, and cosmetics based on their safety for use in people.

Two important amendments have been made to the 1938 law. In 1952, Congress passed the Durham–Humphrey Amendment, which directed FDA to divide drug products into two categories: those that require a prescription and those that may be sold without a prescription. When a prescription is required, these products are sometimes called *legend drugs* because the FDA requires a symbol or statement on the product's packaging. Those agents that do not require prescriptions are called *nonprescription, nonlegend,* or *over-the-counter drugs*. In response to birth defects in Europe caused by thalidomide, Congress later gave FDA more authority by passing the Kefauver–Harris Drug Amendments of 1962. These amendments allowed FDA to control the research into new drugs, to require that new drugs be effective for the conditions listed in product labeling (in addition to being safe), to remove drugs from the market more easily when necessary, and to more easily regulate advertising of prescription drugs.

Drug-Approval Process

FDA's authority to determine which drug products can be marketed in the United States is very broad. A pharmaceutical company that wants to market a product must prove to FDA that the drug is both safe to use in people and effective for the claimed uses. FDA requires evidence from special kinds of research studies called *controlled clinical trials*. In these trials, the pharmaceutical company must compare the new drug with either *placebo* (dosage forms that look like the real product but that contain no active agent) or an alternative agent known to be effective.

Medications going through this FDA premarketing process are called investigational drugs. Pharmaceutical companies collectively spend billions of dollars each year ($55.2 billion in 2006) searching for compounds to test and conducting investigational drug studies. Through chemical and animal studies, company researchers identify a compound they believe will be useful in people. Then the company files with FDA an Investigational New Drug (IND) application. Figure 3-1 shows why this is such an expensive process. For every drug that is eventually approved by FDA, the companies screen 5,000 to 10,000 compounds, and the entire process consumes years of valuable patent life. In addition, according to the Pharmaceutical Research and Manufacturers of America, the average cost of bringing one new drug to the market in the United States averages $802 million (http://www.phrma.org/key_industry_facts_about_phrma/, accessed August 18, 2006).

If FDA approves the IND application, the company begins testing in people. These tests progress through three phases, shown in Figure 3-1:

- **Phase I:** The investigational drug is tested in a small number (20 to 80) of healthy volunteers (people who do not have any active disease) to ensure its safety and to determine appropriate doses in humans during Phase I.
- **Phase II:** A slightly larger number (100 to 300) of patient volunteers (people who have the target disease) use the drug in Phase II to see if it continues to prove safe and to determine if it works.
- **Phase III:** If FDA allows the company to proceed into Phase III tests, the company recruits 1,000 to 5,000 patient volunteers to participate in a controlled clinical trial. These trials are used to test for efficacy as well as to identify adverse effects (harmful and unintended side effects) of the drug during short- and long-term use.

After Phase III trials are complete, the pharmaceutical company reviews the data. If the numbers seem to indicate safety and efficacy of the drug, the company files a New Drug Application (NDA) with FDA. The federal agency can take several months or even years to review the NDA before either approving or denying the application. Even when the NDA is approved, FDA usually requires further post-marketing testing, sometimes called Phase IV, to check for adverse effects that occur in very small percentages of patients taking the drug.

Despite the complexity of this process, some 20 to 50 new drugs come onto the US market each year. With the new knowledge we now have about the *human genome*

As a pharmacy technician, you may encounter patients who are receiving investigational new drugs. Special procedures and record keeping must be followed when handling these agents.

FIGURE 3-1

Drug Development: How Compounds Move from the Laboratory to Clinical Use.

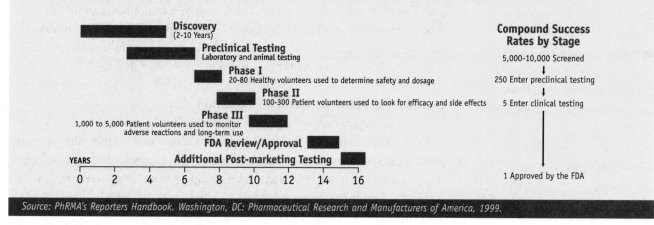

Source: PhRMA's Reporters Handbook. Washington, DC: Pharmaceutical Research and Manufacturers of America, 1999.

(the 46 human chromosomes), companies are expecting to increase both the number and the types of new drugs they are researching. As this happens, pharmacogenomics and pharmacogenetics—the use and dosing of drugs with knowledge of people's genetic make-ups—will increase in frequency and importance.

As a pharmacy technician, you may encounter patients who are receiving investigational new drugs. Especially in large teaching hospitals, your pharmacy may be assisting with numerous drug protocols. Special procedures and record keeping must be followed when handling these agents. For instance, these studies are usually placebo controlled. This means that up to one half of the patients in the study are receiving tablets or capsules that are identical in appearance but have no active drug. By using these placebos, the researchers can measure the improvements in patients' conditions that are attributable to the new drug. The studies are usually also double blinded, which means that neither the researchers nor the patients know who is receiving the active drug and who is getting a placebo. For this purpose, the pharmacy often prepares identical dosage forms (tablets or capsules), some with active drug and some with placebo. If these products were to get mixed up, it could ruin the study. If your responsibilities include investigational agents, be sure that you understand the relevant policies and procedures adopted in your facility.

Drug Withdrawals and Recalls

Despite all the effort to make sure that drugs are safe and effective before they come onto the market, serious or fatal adverse effects sometimes occur after a medication is used widely. Even when a drug is tested in a few thousand people, rare but serious side effects may not become apparent (or even occur) until millions of people are exposed to the drug. When these situations develop, the drug product is withdrawn from the market either temporarily or permanently. While the withdrawals are often termed voluntary, the companies usually act after they and FDA officials conclude that the risk of continued use of the drug outweighs the possible benefits of keeping the agent on the market.

FDA also sometimes asks companies to recall specific batches, or lots, of their products. The reasons for recalls vary from serious situations, such as products that contain the wrong drug or too much of the correct drug, to less important situations, such as the company's manufacturing processes have been called into question, but nothing is necessarily wrong with the drug products.

To place recalls into perspective, FDA divides them into three types, as shown in Table 3-1.

As a pharmacy technician, you will no doubt be called on to find the affected lots of recalled drug products. These recalls are announced by the companies and publicized by FDA on its web site at www.fda.gov/opacom/7alerts.html. If an investigational drug or a radiopharmaceutical (see Chapter 10) is recalled, special conditions may apply to the return, handling, or destruction of these medicinals; be sure to follow the policies and procedures of your workplace in such cases (see Chapter 15).

Dietary Supplement Health Education Act

Because consumers are bombarded by much false and misleading information about health foods, alternative medicines, and dietary supplements, pharmacists and pharmacy technicians can play an important role in helping patients sort out legitimate, useful products from those that are just quackery. The first step in providing this help is to understand the rules governing the available products and the role FDA plays in the system.

TABLE 3-1

Three Types of Recalls Classified by the FDA

- **Class I:** Continued use of the product is very likely to cause serious adverse effects or deaths in people.

- **Class II:** Use of the product could cause temporary but reversible effects or there is little chance that serious adverse effects would result from use of the product.

- **Class III:** Use of the recalled lots or product is unlikely to cause adverse effects in people.

In 1994, the U.S. Congress passed an important bill, the Dietary Supplement Health Education Act of 1994 (DSHEA), which governs the sale and marketing of dietary supplements. Also known as alternative medicines, vitamins, minerals, herbs, or amino acids, these products are in a gray area between regular foods and medications.

As a result of this bill, products labeled as dietary supplements may make three types of claims on their labels, as shown in Table 3-2.

FDA, in implementing DSHEA, required that dietary supplements carry a "Supplement Facts" panel, similar to the "Nutrition Facts" panel you see on most foods. The supplements panel includes the following:

- An appropriate serving size
- Information on 14 nutrients, when present at significant levels, including sodium, vitamin A, vitamin C, calcium, and iron
- The presence of other vitamins and minerals if they are added or are part of the product's nutritional claims
- Dietary ingredients for which no Reference Daily Intakes have been established
- For proprietary blends of ingredients (for example, a mixture of herbs for the liver), the names of the ingredients and the total amount of ingredients (the specific amount of each ingredient is not required)

A key point with regard to dietary supplements is that they are not reviewed and regulated by FDA in the same way as drugs. For instance, for a drug to be marketed in the United States, a sponsoring company must prove to FDA that the drug is both safe and effective. In contrast, dietary supplement companies must merely notify FDA at least 75 days before a product is to go on the market. FDA can only stop the company from marketing if the agency can prove that the product is not safe (efficacy is not considered with dietary supplements). So, in terms of both FDA process and the onus of responsibility, dietary supplements are the opposite of drugs. That is, with drugs, manufacturers of drugs must convince FDA that new medications are safe and effective before they are allowed to market products containing that agent; with dietary supplements, FDA must prove lack of safety in order to stop a manufacturer from marketing a product, and it has only 75 days to do so. In addition, manufacturing processes are not nearly as strict with dietary supplements as with drug products.

TABLE 3-2

Three Types of Claims Made by Dietary Supplements

- Nutrient-content claims describe the amounts of nutrients contained in the product. Examples include "High in calcium" or "Excellent source of vitamin C."

- Disease claims, which must be based on established scientific evidence, describe well-established links between diet and health. Examples include prevention of certain types of birth defects by folic acid supplements and prevention of osteoporosis by calcium supplements.

- Nutrition support claims describe relationships between dietary intake and disease or health, such as the use of vitamin C in preventing scurvy. They may include "structure-function claims," such as "calcium builds strong bones" or "antioxidants maintain cell integrity."

Third Class of Medications

A perpetual issue at the FDA is a proposed third class of drugs that could be prescribed and dispensed by pharmacists. In the United States, drugs are currently divided into two classes: those that require a prescription from an authorized prescriber and those that can be sold without a prescription (i.e., over-the-counter or nonprescription medications). Several other industrialized countries—including Canada, New Zealand, the United Kingdom, and Australia—have a third class of medications, ones that do not require a prescription but can only be obtained from a pharmacist.

Since 1974, various professional pharmacy organizations have petitioned the FDA for the establishment of a third class of drugs. Advocates contend that such a move would increase pharmacist interaction with consumers, thereby leading to safer use of OTC medicines. With a growing number of agents becoming available without a prescription (referred to as the Rx-to-OTC shift), an increased degree of pharmacist involvement in the use of nonprescription medications is warranted.

As this text was being prepared, FDA approved a politically controversial Rx-to-OTC switch, involving the morning-after pills that are used for emergency contraception. Because of moral, ethical, legal, and political concerns, FDA approved the switch only for women aged 18 and older, and in a historic decision, left levonorgestrel (Plan B—Duramed) prescription-only for younger girls. Pharmacists will be the gatekeepers in this situation, stocking the product "behind the counter" and providing it without a prescription to older patients and as a prescription product to younger ones.

During the APhA 2007 meeting, FDA announced that it is taking a close look at the development of regulatory processes for a third class of drugs. While FDA has previously maintained it had no legal authority to approve a drug only for a third class of drugs, it does have the authority to place controls on how a drug is distributed and handled. This announcement indicates that FDA may consider using the experience gained with Plan B to either seek Congressional action that would create a third class of drugs or might consider making other agents available under restrictions similar to those for Plan B.

Opponents to the third class of drugs generally include physician and nursing groups, manufacturers of nonprescription agents and dietary supplements (represented by the trade association, Consumer Healthcare Products Association [www.chpa-info.org]), as well as the U.S. Government Accountability Office (GAO). While not specifically referring to emergency contraception, these groups and organizations believe that in general placing products in a pharmacist-only category would be inconvenient for consumers, limit the consumer's choice of product, and cause price increases.

Centers for Medicare & Medicaid Services

The Centers for Medicare & Medicaid Services (CMS) is the current name for the agency that administers federal coverage of health care. It was known as the Health Care Financing Administration (HCFA) from its inception during the Great Society phase of the Lyndon B. Johnson Administration (1965) until it was renamed during the George W. Bush Administration in 2001.

While the Medicare and Medicaid programs are very complicated, one can think of the Medicare program as paying for acute (hospital) care for the elderly and the Medicaid program as covering the indigent (those without insurance or enough money to pay for care on their own). Until 2006, Medicare paid for prescription drugs only when they were used in an acute-care institution (hospital) or in conjunction with certain medical devices such as in-dwelling catheters (tubes that go into very large veins of the body). Beginning in 2006, a Part D was added to the Medicare benefit that pays for prescription drugs for all beneficiaries (see Chapter 6 for more background on the emergence of this new benefit). Medicaid pays for outpatient prescription drugs and other care for indigent patients in community pharmacies, nursing homes, or hospitals. Some people qualify under both Medicare and Medicaid, and they are termed "dual eligibles."

Important to note is that the Medicaid program is financed jointly by the federal and state governments, with each contributing about one half of the funds. Thus, though Medicaid is a federal program, pharmacists' interactions are usually with the agency within the state government that coordinates the program. As state budgets have been squeezed more and more recently, the Medicaid programs have been increasingly tightened. The effects of these economic constraints have been severe in many states. For example, Medicaid patients' prescriptions often must be filled off a state-approved drug list (or "formulary"), recipients may be limited to a certain number of prescriptions per month, and states have sometimes held up Medicaid payments for several months because of budgetary shortfall.

Likewise, even though Medicare Part D is a federal program, it is administered through dozens of private prescription drug providers, or PDPs. Every PDP has its own formulary, and Medicare beneficiaries can choose any PDP operating in their geographic area (usually a state). Pharmacists' interactions are generally with these intermediaries when it comes to obtaining reimbursement for prescriptions and getting approval for nonformulary medications.

The Medicare Part D program also included a provision for medication therapy management (MTM) services. During the first year of the program, PDPs were required to provide, either directly or through pharmacies, MTM services to those Medicare patients who were being treated for multiple diseases with multiple medications and who were expected to need at least $4,000 worth of medications during the year. Just how pharmacies and PDPs met this requirement is not yet clear, as efforts during this year focused more on the drug-distribution aspects of the new program. In the long run, CMS has stated that MTM services should become the "cornerstone" of Medicare Part D, and the associated payment aspect could enable pharmacists to further develop their pharmaceutical care and clinical pharmacy services for elderly patients. If this happens, the pharmacy technician's role in processing and preparing prescription medications will become even more important than it is today.

In addition to the daily requirements associated with processing individual prescriptions, pharmacies must comply with certain broader requirements mandated by CMS and/or state agencies. These are called "conditions of participation" because providers—including hospitals, physicians, nursing homes, and pharmacies—must agree to them in order to participate in the Medicare and Medicaid programs. Conditions for participation specify many operational, procedural, and outcome details, and you may see that your pharmacy is changing a procedure or getting a new type of hood for making intravenous fluids because of such requirements.

Drug Enforcement Administration

All medications are dangerous enough to merit special approval by FDA, but some agents require even more scrutiny and controls. Drugs or chemicals with a potential for abuse or for physical or psychological addiction are called *controlled substances*. (*Addictive drugs*, such as heroin, are those that, used once by a person, can produce physical or psychological symptoms if use is not continued.) These agents are regulated by DEA, which is a part of the US Department of Justice. Some of these drugs—such as heroin and marijuana—are illegal in the United States. Other controlled substances that have accepted medical uses can be marketed, but their label must prominently display a large letter C and a Roman numeral of their class (see Table 3-3) to show that they are subject to special regulations.

History

As social problems with drug abuse reached epidemic proportions in the late 1960s, Congress responded in 1970 by passing the Comprehensive Drug Abuse Prevention and Control Act and the Controlled Substances Act. These laws created the DEA, giving it responsibility for both regulating the medical use of addictive drugs and fighting the illicit drug trafficking problem. DEA agents thus have two different roles: one in which they fight those who are smuggling and selling illegal drugs and another in which they apprehend health care professionals who are breaking laws, or diverting legal drugs into the illegal market, or both.

TABLE 3-3

Categories of Regulation for Controlled Substances

- **Schedule I** drugs have high abuse and addiction potential and have no accepted medical use in the United States. Examples include heroin, LSD, marijuana, and mescaline.

- **Schedule II** drugs have high abuse and addiction potential but do have medical applications. Examples include cocaine, Dilaudid (hydromorphone), Ritalin (methylphenidate), Seconal (secobarbital), and several types of amphetamines ("diet pills" or "speed").

- **Schedule III** drugs have abuse and addiction potential but not as much as those in Schedule II. Examples include Tylenol #3 (acetaminophen with codeine) and Fastin (phentermine).

- **Schedule IV** drugs have a low potential for abuse. Examples include Valium (diazepam), Halcion (triazolam), and Darvon (propoxyphene).

- **Schedule V** drugs have low abuse potential and have very limited amounts of drugs in each dosage form. Examples are Lomotil (diphenoxylate and atropine) and some cough syrups containing codeine. Some Schedule V products do not even require a prescription (because of FDA regulations), but they must be dispensed by a pharmacist because of DEA rules.

Controlled Substance Regulations

DEA has the authority to specify which drugs need special controls. These drugs are defined in five categories of controlled substances, as shown in Table 3-3.

DEA requires that pharmacies keep meticulous records about the controlled substances they stock. Through the pharmacist-in-charge, the pharmacy must be able to account for every dose of Schedule II controlled substances and keep a perpetual inventory (an ongoing record) that DEA can inspect at any time. In addition, DEA requires that a manual inventory (actually counting every tablet, capsule, and injection) be performed every 2 years, usually on May 1 of odd-numbered years. Similar records based on approximate counts of Schedule III, IV, and V drugs must be kept.

Because of the special care required in ordering controlled substances and keeping records about them, pharmacy technicians often assist with these processes in pharmacies with large inventories, such as those in hospitals. DEA order form 222 (Figure 3-2), supplied in triplicate but also now available electronically, is used for ordering Schedule II controlled substances. In pharmacies still using manual order forms, the three copies are processed as follows:

- Copies 1 and 2 are sent to the supplier, usually a drug wholesaler but sometimes the drug manufacturer.
- Copy 3 is filed at the pharmacy.

When the order is received, copy 3 of the DEA form 222 is pulled. The pharmacist processing the order should record on copy 3 the date and amount of drug product received. Copy 3 is then refiled and kept for 2 years.

The electronic version of form 222 has been designed to ensure confidentiality of communications, authentication of the sending party, integrity of communications (the recipient can tell if the order was changed in transit), and nonrepudiation (using DEA-supplied electronic signatures that are difficult to forge). Electronic records supporting each transaction must be retained for 2 years, similar to the paper copies of Form 222, and suppliers are required to report transactions to DEA within 2 business days.[1]

Technicians working in community pharmacies need to take care with prescriptions for controlled substances, especially those in Schedule II. Most forged prescriptions are for controlled substances. When receiving a prescription calling for one of these agents, the technicians should first verify the patient's name and get his or her address, a DEA requirement. If anything about the prescription looks unusual, a pharmacist should be alerted quietly but immediately. Forged prescriptions may:

- Have altered quantities
- Be written on prescription forms that were stolen or photocopied
- Be written on prescription forms from hospitals (which do not have a specific physician's name)
- Be written on prescription forms from distant cities or even another state

FIGURE 3-2

DEA Order Form.

	See Reverse of PURCHASER'S Copy for Instructions	No order form may be issued for Schedule I and II substances unless a completed application form has been received. (21 CFR 1305.04).	OMB APPROVAL No. 1117-0010

TO: *(Name of Supplier)* | **STREET ADDRESS**

	CITY and STATE		DATE	NATIONAL DRUG CODE	TO BE FILLED IN BY PURCHASER	
Line No.	No. of Packages	Size of Packages	Name of Item (TO BE FILLED IN BY PURCHASER)		No. of Packages Received	Date Received
1						
2						
3						
4						
5						
6						
7						
8						
9						
10						

◄ **LAST LINE COMPLETED** *(MUST BE 10 OR LESS)* | **SIGNATURE OF PURCHASER OR ATTORNEY OR AGENT**

Date Issued	DEA Registration No.	Name and Address of Registrant
Schedules		
Registered as a	No. of this Order Form	

DEA Form-222 (Oct. 1992)

U.S. OFFICIAL ORDER FORMS - SCHEDULES I & II
DRUG ENFORCEMENT ADMINISTRATION
PURCHASER'S Copy 3

Source: Pharmacy Technician Certification Board. Accessed at http://www.ptcb.org/About/statistics.aspx, June 23, 2006.

The prescriber's name, address, and DEA number must be on the prescription. DEA numbers should be verified for new prescribers using the following procedure:

- Check DEA number to be sure it has two letters and seven numbers (e.g., AA9999999).
- Add up the first, third, and fifth digits, and record the result as SUM1.
- Add up the second, fourth, and sixth digits, multiply the result times 2, and record the result as SUM2.
- Add SUM1 to SUM2 to obtain SUM3.

In valid DEA numbers, the seventh digit will be the second digit of SUM3. If it is not, then the DEA number is not valid.

For example, the DEA number AP1857397 can be checked as follows:

- Two letters and seven digits are present.
- The sum of the first, third, and fifth digits is 9 (SUM1).
- The sum of the second, fourth, and sixth digits is 24, and twice this amount is 48 (SUM2).
- The sum of 48 and 9 is 57 (SUM3; second digit is 7).
- The seventh digit of the DEA number is 7, so the number is legitimate.

If a prescription appears altered, you and the pharmacist should follow your pharmacy's policy about what steps to take. For prescriptions you know to be altered, you might call local police or authorities while trying to get the person who presented the prescription to

If a prescription appears altered, you and the pharmacist should follow your pharmacy's policy about what steps to take.

An important role

of pharmacists is to

ensure that patients

understand what

drugs they are

taking, what each

drug is for,

and how each drug

is to be taken.

remain in the pharmacy. If you are fairly certain the prescription is forged, but you are not positive, pharmacy policy might call for you to refuse to fill the prescription. Depending on the policy and the circumstances, you may or may not return the apparently forged prescription to the presenter. This situation is quite serious; the presenter, if addicted to the drug, may be desperate to get it and could react violently. If you refuse to return a legitimate prescription, you, the pharmacist, and the pharmacy might be sued by the presenter. The pharmacist should determine the action to be taken, considering his or her own assessment of the situation and personal beliefs and the company's or pharmacy's policy.

A final area of concern about controlled substances is what to do when the drugs expire or get too old to use. As with all drug products, controlled substances have expiration dates on each package. Once these dates pass, the product should not be dispensed. However, because of the need to account for all controlled substances to the DEA, the pharmacy cannot just destroy these agents. Again, you should follow company or pharmacy policy regarding the disposition of controlled substances. Generally, certain DEA forms must be completed, and two or more licensed individuals must witness the destruction of the controlled substances. Similar procedures may apply in hospitals or nursing homes when controlled substances are returned to the pharmacy after patients are discharged or die.

TABLE 3-4

Information a Pharmacist Must Discuss with Patients

Under OBRA '90, a pharmacist is required to discuss the following information with the patient or caregiver:

- Name and description of the medication
- Dosage form, dose, route of administration, and duration of drug therapy
- Special directions and precautions for preparation, administration, and use of the medication
- Common or severe side effects, adverse reactions, or interactions and therapeutic contraindications that may be encountered, including ways of avoiding them, and the action required if they occur
- Techniques for self monitoring of drug therapy
- Proper storage
- Prescription refill information
- Action to be taken in the event of a missed dose

Federal Patient Information Initiatives

An important role of pharmacists is to ensure that patients understand what drugs they are taking, what each drug is for, and how each drug is to be taken. Some drugs taken by mouth should be taken on an empty stomach, while others must be taken with food. Patients often need to learn how to use specialized administration devices such as inhalers or to give injections of drugs such as insulin.

Because of the importance of pharmacists in educating patients, during the 1990s the federal government sought to ensure that this information would be conveyed to patients through two actions: OBRA '90 and FDA's Medication Guide Program.

Omnibus Budget Reconciliation Act of 1990

In 1990, Congress passed OBRA '90. Among its other provisions, the bill required that pharmacists offer to counsel patients whose prescriptions were being paid for under Medicaid, one of two major federal health-reimbursement plans. The bill also required state Medicaid administrators, who oversee the programs, to conduct reviews of the drug use in each state to ensure drugs are used as optimally as possible.

The implications of OBRA '90 for technicians are twofold. First, because the counseling requirement was added to state regulations by most state boards of pharmacy, all patients should be offered pharmacist counseling. If a patient asks for counseling, notify a pharmacist. Under OBRA '90, the pharmacist is required to discuss with the patient or caregiver the information shown in Table 3-4.

In addition, the pharmacist is required under OBRA '90 to record and maintain the information shown in Table 3-5.

Second, the drug-use review requirement is typically done in real-time by computer. This means that while technicians are entering prescription orders into the pharmacy's computer, various alerts may pop up on the computer screen notifying the pharmacist of drug interactions, clinical problems, or reimbursement problems. The technician will need to refer many of these alerts to the pharmacist for a decision about whether to dispense the prescription, talk with the patient, or contact the prescriber.

Food and Drug Administration's Medication Guide Program

For a quarter century, FDA has been looking for an effective way to ensure the provision of patient information when prescription drugs are dispensed by pharmacists. The agency finally succeeded in this effort in 1999, despite the opposition of pharmacy, medicine, and the pharmaceutical industry.

FDA ruled that it could require manufacturer-produced medication guides for any drug product under any one of the following conditions:

- The drug is one for which patient information could help prevent serious adverse effects.
- The drug has serious risks relative to benefits.
- The drug is important to health, and patient adherence to directions for use is crucial to the drug's effectiveness.

When FDA issued this rule, 70% of patients were already receiving some type of written information from pharmacists at the time medicines were provided. Recognizing this reality, FDA signaled that it intends to only occasionally require medication guides, at least early on, and that these guides would be required only in cases of new drugs when they are first marketed in the United States. In addition, legislation passed in 1996 requires evaluation of the frequency and quality of patient information given to patients by pharmacists. If certain benchmarks (acceptable levels) are not met by 2006, FDA is empowered to issue further regulations to ensure that patients have access to the information they need to use their medicines safely and effectively. The coming years will tell whether pharmacy has met the challenge or will be required to do so under FDA's purview.

In the meantime, you will need to provide medication guides, or MedGuides as they are called, to the patient when they have been mandated, and your pharmacy's computer system may generate leaflets for other drugs. Follow developments in this area to stay up-to-date on which products have mandatory medication guides. Publications such as the American Pharmacists Association's *Pharmacy Today* and *Drug Topics* carry articles on such news stories, and an index to drug-specific information can be accessed on the FDA web site (http://www.fda.gov/cder/drug/DrugSafety/DrugIndex.htm).

Americans with Disabilities Act

According to the US Department of Justice, some 50 million Americans have disabilities of one type or another, including about one half of those older than age 65—the very population that uses about two-thirds of medications. These can range from severe physical problems that confine people to wheelchairs to psychological disabilities that must be compensated for in schoolrooms and testing situations. Whatever the nature of the disability, the Americans with Disabilities Act (ADA) prescribes various actions that must be taken by employers and businesses throughout the United States.

Within pharmacies, ADA requirements may be as simple as elimination of barriers such as steps or narrow doors or aisles that cannot be navigated by people in wheelchairs to as complicated as accommodating the needs of an employee with a speech, hearing, or visual disability. Particularly difficult is counseling of patients with disabilities, as they may not be able to read inserts provided with prescriptions or understand what pharmacists are saying

TABLE 3-5

Information Pharmacists Must Record and Maintain

Under OBRA '90 pharmacists are required to record and maintain the following information:

- Patient's name, address, telephone number, date of birth (or age), and sex
- Patient's individual history when important, including diseases, known allergies and drug reactions, and a comprehensive list of medications and relevant medical devices
- Pharmacist's comments about the individual's drug therapy

You will need to provide medication guides, or MedGuides as they are called, to the patient when they have been mandated, and your pharmacy's computer system may generate leaflets for other drugs.

TABLE 3-6

When Pharmacists Counsel Patients with Disabilities

Key points to remember when counseling patients with disabilities include:

- People with disabilities don't want to be treated any differently from anyone else. Offer help if they ask for it, but otherwise treat them as you would any other patient in the pharmacy.

- Remember that service animals, such as seeing-eye dogs, must be allowed in the pharmacy and other health facilities.

- Special labeling, such as Braille, is not required for products in the store. You should read the labels to blind patients as they request it.

- More information about ADA is available from www.ada.gov; 800/514-0301 (voice); 800/514-0383 (TTY).

about the proper use of their medications. Talk with the pharmacists and managers in your pharmacy about what steps have been taken to comply with the ADA—and about any areas that could be improved in this regard. Some key points to remember are summarized in Table 3-6.

State Boards of Pharmacy

The division of responsibilities between the state and federal governments follows the line of reasoning known as states' rights: all responsibilities not specifically assigned to the federal government in the United States Constitution are reserved for the states. Drug and pharmacy regulation is not mentioned in the Constitution and is therefore delegated to the states. However, this has been an area in which the federal government has creatively enlarged its role when it believed that public health was at risk. In fact, the current development of Internet-based pharmacies is creating a need for action by federal authorities, because states have difficulty regulating pharmacies located in other states. But, for now, states remain the main regulatory authority for pharmacies, pharmacists, and technicians.

States regulate professions through *boards* composed largely of members of the profession with a smaller number of consumer members. Federal laws generally do not specifically deal with regulation of the professions; as mentioned earlier, FDA's legend drugs do not specify what types of practitioners may legally prescribe these drugs. Federal law often depends heavily on the framework present in states.

State boards of pharmacy developed around 1900 after their organization was proposed in model pharmacy laws developed by the American Pharmaceutical (now Pharmacists) Association. Pharmacy organizations and pharmacy laws have often grown together, and the organization of the state boards followed this trend. However, it is important to remember that state boards of pharmacy have as their primary mission the protection of the public from the profession—not vice versa. Pharmacy associations, conversely, exist to promote the profession, which sometimes leads them along paths that are not necessarily in the overall public interest.

State boards of pharmacy, based on authority granted to them by the various state legislatures, promulgate the specific regulations that govern the practice of pharmacy on a day-to-day basis. Boards issue licenses to pharmacists and pharmacies. Sometimes they register or license technicians. Boards specify by what mechanisms pharmacists, and sometimes technicians, can keep their licenses in force. They have investigative arms that police the profession, and they are the judge and jury for pharmacists (and, in some states, technicians) who violate state pharmacy laws. The decisions rendered by the state board of pharmacy can drastically affect the way in which the profession is practiced in a given state.

The National Association of Boards of Pharmacy (NABP) was formed in 1904. It has grown to a powerful position in coordinating activities among the state boards. It now provides a national examination, called the NAPLEX® (North American Pharmacist Licensure Examination™), for administration in all states. NABP coordinates the reciprocation of pharmacist licenses between states. The association develops model pharmacy practice acts that state legislatures can consider for updating state laws to incorporate changes in pharmacy. NABP also certifies Internet pharmacies as having met minimum criteria that indicate that their activities are within federal and state laws.

It is impossible to convey the specifics of each state's pharmacy board regulations in a national text; you will need to become familiar with the rules in the states in which you work. Talk with your employer or the pharmacists with whom you work about what you need to know. You may also contact your state board directly for information.

Voluntary Accreditation Programs

In addition to legal requirements for practicing pharmacy, pharmacists and pharmacies often voluntarily participate in other types of oversight programs. For instance, they may choose to train pharmacy residents, and this opens up the pharmacy to inspection by national accrediting bodies for residency programs. A hospital may want to be reimbursed through certain federal or private payers, and these organizations may require accreditation through CMS or voluntary alternatives. In all these situations, surveyors visit the hospital or pharmacy and assess its compliance with certain standards of practice, care, and quality.

The major accrediting body in health care is the Joint Commission on Accreditation of Healthcare Organizations. The Joint Commission is a nongovernmental body. Because Joint Commission accreditation can take the place of visits by CMS officials for providers such as hospitals and clinical laboratories, the Joint Commission visit becomes a major focal point. The Joint Commission has begun some pharmacy-specific accreditation activities, especially in long-term care.

Accreditation of residency and training programs and the certification of individual practitioners for increased knowledge in pharmacy specialty areas are increasingly important in pharmacy. The following are examples of voluntary oversight by the profession.

Accreditation of Training Programs

Most people are familiar with the process by which physicians enter residency programs after graduation to specialize in various medical specialty areas. But few people realize that many pharmacy graduates enter residency programs too. At some schools, one third to one half of pharmacy graduates go on to this type of specialized training. This trend has increased as a result of pharmacy shifting to the doctor of pharmacy, or PharmD, as the entry-level degree. In addition, the number of community pharmacy residencies is growing, further increasing the proportion of graduating student pharmacists who complete a residency before taking a "real" job.

Pharmacy residencies developed first in hospital pharmacy in the 1930s (they were called internships until 1962), and residencies in hospitals are still the most common. The American Society of Health-System Pharmacists (ASHP) began accrediting hospital pharmacy residencies in 1963, and it currently recognizes more than 800 programs in a wide variety of pharmacy practice settings, including traditional hospitals, community pharmacies, and managed care organizations. ASHP eliminated the terminology "hospital pharmacy residency" and "clinical pharmacy residency" in 1992; all are now recognized as pharmacy practice residencies or simply pharmacy residencies. ASHP offers several types of specialized residencies. In 1999, it began accrediting managed care pharmacy residencies with the Academy of Managed Care Pharmacy and community pharmacy residencies with the American Pharmaceutical (now Pharmacists) Association.

In 2003, the Society reorganized its accreditation standards into a postgraduate year 1 (PGY1) and year 2 (PGY2). PGY1 programs can be conducted at one or more sites, and colleges of pharmacy can participate as sponsoring organizations. Residents learn about managing and improving the medication-use process, providing evidence-based, patient-centered medication therapy management with interdisciplinary teams, exercising leadership and practice management skills, demonstrating project management skills, providing medication and practice-related education/training, and using medical informatics.[2]

Most people are familiar with the process by which physicians enter residency programs after graduation to specialize in various medical specialty areas. But few people realize that many pharmacy graduates enter residency programs too.

PGY2 pharmacy residency programs focus on a specific area of practice, such as primary care/ambulatory, critical care, drug information, geriatrics, oncology, psychiatric, or internal medicine.[3]

ASHP also accredits technician training programs. As described briefly in Chapter 1, accredited technician training programs are based chiefly in community colleges or technical schools, but some hospitals and colleges of pharmacy also have such programs. In late 2006, ASHP recognized more than 90 accredited technician training programs, 91% of which were in community colleges or vocational/technical colleges.[4]

Certification of Individuals

Certification is a term that is becoming increasingly common in pharmacy, particularly for pharmacists who practice in highly specialized areas and for pharmacy technicians. Certification is a form of self-discipline or self-control by a profession, and the process works when employers and health care professionals are able to police themselves. For instance, any physician can legally perform brain surgery, but only those who are certified by a medical specialty board as neurosurgeons generally do so. If a substantial number of noncertified physicians began offering services they were unqualified to perform, the state would likely step in and set up a licensure mechanism. Thus, a process of self-regulation protects the public health and eliminates the need for governmental action.

For the profession of pharmacy, a Board of Pharmaceutical Specialties (BPS) was organized in 1976 to recognize the activities in pharmacy that required certification and to develop processes to accomplish that certification. Since then, it has recognized five specialties[5], as shown in Table 3-7.

BPS has also recognized two subspecialties to pharmacotherapy, infectious diseases and cardiology. More subspecialties, called "Added Qualifications" in BPS parlance, will be considered by BPS in the future.[6]

The purpose of pharmacy certification is to demonstrate personal achievement in these specialized areas. Employers also often require applicants to have certain credentials, including certification status in these specialty areas.

Pharmacy technicians are also becoming certified. For you, certification is a way to demonstrate accomplishment in a career that has no uniform educational or training requirements and to demonstrate to employers a given level of knowledge about the activities of pharmacy technicians. The Pharmacy Technician Certification Board (PTCB) is the certifying body for pharmacy technicians. At the end of 2005, PTCB's 10th anniversary, nearly 284,000 candidates had taken the Pharmacy Technician Certification Examination (PTCE), and 79% of them had passed the test and been recognized as Certified Pharmacy Technicians (CPhTs). With 6,700 CPhTs whose certification was transferred from state examinations given before PTCB was formed, the total number of CPhTs exceeds 250,000 at the end of 2006, with some states boasting large numbers of CPhTs as a result of state laws and regulations.[7] State boards of pharmacy are increasingly requiring that those assisting in the preparation of prescriptions be CPhTs. In states without such laws and regulations, employers use certification of technicians to determine a technician's readiness for promotions into certain jobs, such as those in intravenous admixture rooms or those that require supervising other technicians.

For more information, access the PTCB Web site at www.ptcb.org or contact the organization at 1100 15th St. NW, Suite 730, Washington, DC 20005-1707; 800-363-8012.

TABLE 3-7

BPS Categories of Specialization

The BPS has recognized five categories of specialization in pharmacy:

- Nuclear pharmacy
- Pharmacotherapy
- Nutrition support pharmacy
- Psychiatric pharmacy
- Oncology pharmacy

Material Safety Data Sheets

While the Occupational Safety and Health Administration (OSHA) has historically been concerned primarily with workplaces with unusual dangers, such as factories or mines, it has recently paid health care settings an increasing amount of attention. A major reason for this scrutiny is an OSHA requirement that information be quickly available about hazardous chemicals stored in the workplace, including pharmacies, hospitals, nursing homes, and other institutions. OSHA categorizes some drugs as hazardous chemicals, which is how pharmacy personnel become involved.[8]

OSHA, a unit in the US Department of Labor, requires that worksites where hazardous chemicals are used or stored do the following:

- Identify and list hazardous chemicals
- Obtain information, in the form of MSDSs, about hazardous chemicals from manufacturers, importers, or distributors of the chemicals
- Develop and implement a written hazard communication program, including labels on the products, MSDSs, and employee training
- When necessitated by spills or employee exposure, communicate hazard information to employees

OSHA defines hazardous chemicals as those that can cause physical damage (such as those that can catch fire or explode) and those that pose a danger to health. Chemicals used or stored in pharmacies may be flammable or explosive, falling into the first category. Several drugs fall into the latter category, including many agents used to treat cancer.

As a pharmacy technician, you will need to know how these OSHA requirements have been addressed in your pharmacy and what to do if an emergency occurs. Talk with your supervisor if this information was not covered in orientation sessions when you were first hired.

Codes of Ethics

At the individual level, the actions of pharmacists and technicians are guided by Codes of Ethics. These statements, approved by national organizations of pharmacists and technicians, help guide behaviors that are not necessarily illegal but that nonetheless may bring harm to the patient.

The Codes of Ethics for pharmacists and technicians are shown in Figures 3-3 and 3-4. Read these documents and talk with your colleagues about them. They are important statements of what you, as a pharmacy technician, should and should not do in your workplace.

Conclusion

Before we get to the processing of prescriptions, you will need to understand the classifications of drugs. Let's move on to Chapter 4!

For More Information

If you are preparing for the Pharmacy Technician Certification Examination and feel that you need more information about the topics discussed in this chapter, consider accessing the Web sites listed in the References for more information.

FIGURE 3-3

Code of Ethics of the American Pharmacists Association.

PREAMBLE: Pharmacists are health professionals who assist individuals in making the best use of medications. This Code, prepared and supported by pharmacists, is intended to state publicly the principles that form the fundamental basis of the roles and responsibilities of pharmacists. These principles, based on moral obligations and virtues, are established to guide pharmacists in relationships with patients, health professionals, and society.

I. *A pharmacist respects the covenantal relationship between the patient and pharmacist.*
Considering the patient-pharmacist relationship as a covenant means that a pharmacist has moral obligations in response to the gift of trust received from society. In return for this gift, a pharmacist promises to help individuals achieve optimum benefit from their medications, to be committed to their welfare, and to maintain their trust.

II. *A pharmacist promotes the good of every patient in a caring, compassionate, and confidential manner.*
A pharmacist places concern for the well-being of the patient at the center of professional practice. In doing so, a pharmacist considers needs stated by the patient as well as those defined by health science. A pharmacist is dedicated to protecting the dignity of the patient. With a caring attitude and a compassionate spirit, a pharmacist focuses on serving the patient in a private and confidential manner.

III. *A pharmacist respects the autonomy and dignity of each patient.*
A pharmacist promotes the right of self-determination and recognizes individual self-worth by encouraging patients to participate in decisions about their health. A pharmacist communicates with patients in terms that are understandable. In all cases, a pharmacist respects personal and cultural differences among patients.

IV. *A pharmacist acts with honesty and integrity in professional relationships.*
A pharmacist has a duty to tell the truth and to act with conviction of conscience. A pharmacist avoids discriminatory practices, behavior or work conditions that impair professional judgment, and actions that compromise dedication to the best interests of patients.

V. *A pharmacist maintains professional competence.*
A pharmacist has a duty to maintain knowledge and abilities as new medications, devices, and technologies become available and as health information advances.

VI. *A pharmacist respects the values and abilities of colleagues and other health professionals.*
When appropriate, a pharmacist asks for the consultation of colleagues or other health professionals or refers the patient. A pharmacist acknowledges that colleagues and other health professionals may differ in the beliefs and values they apply to the care of the patient.

VII. *A pharmacist serves individual, community, and societal needs.*
The primary obligation of a pharmacist is to individual patients. However, the obligations of a pharmacist may at times extend beyond the individual to the community and society. In these situations, the pharmacist recognizes the responsibilities that accompany these obligations and acts accordingly.

VIII. *A pharmacist seeks justice in the distribution of health resources.*
When health resources are allocated, a pharmacist is fair and equitable, balancing the needs of patients and society.

Adopted by the membership of the American Pharmaceutical (now Pharmacists) Association, October 27, 1994.

Code of Ethics for Pharmacy Technicians.

PREAMBLE: Pharmacy technicians are health care professionals who assist pharmacists in providing the best possible care for patients. The principles of this code, which apply to pharmacy technicians working in any and all settings, are based on the application and support of the moral obligations that guide the pharmacy profession in relationships with patients, health care professionals, and society.

PRINCIPLES

A pharmacy technician's first consideration is to ensure the health and safety of the patient and to use knowledge and skills to the best of his/her ability in serving others.

A PHARMACY TECHNICIAN

- supports and promotes honesty and integrity in the profession, which includes a duty to observe the law, maintain the highest moral and ethical conduct at all times, and uphold the ethical principles of the profession;

- assists and supports the pharmacist in the safe, efficacious, and cost-effective distribution of health services and health care resources;

- respects and values the abilities of pharmacists, colleagues, and other health care professionals;

- maintains competency in his/her practice and continually enhances his/her professional knowledge and expertise;

- respects and supports the patient's individuality, dignity, and confidentiality;

- respects the confidentiality of a patient's records and discloses pertinent information only with proper authorization;

- never assists in the dispensing, promoting, or distribution of medications or medical devices that are not of good quality or do not meet the standards required by law;

- does not engage in any activity that will discredit the profession and will expose, without fear or favor, illegal or unethical conduct in the profession; and

- associates with and engages in the support of organizations which promote the profession of pharmacy through the utilization and enhancement of pharmacy technicians.

*For you,
certification is a way
to demonstrate
accomplishment in a
career that has no
uniform educational
or training
requirements and to
demonstrate to
employers a given
level of knowledge
about the activities
of pharmacy
technicians.*

References

1. Drug Enforcement Administration. Electronic Orders for Controlled Substances and Notice of Meeting; Final Rule and Notice. Fed Regist. 2005(Apr 1);70(62):16901–19. http://frwebgate4.access.gpo.gov

2. American Society of Health-System Pharmacists. Accessed at http://www.ashp.org/rtp/index.cfm, September 3, 2006.

3. American Society of Health-System Pharmacists. Accessed at http://www.ashp.org/rtp/PDF/FAQ_newSTD.pdf, September 3, 2006.

4. Written communication, Janet L. Teeters, MS, of the American Society of Health-System Pharmacists, September 8, 2006.

5. Anonymous. Board of Pharmaceutical Specialties: over 20 years of service to the public and the pharmacy profession. Accessed at http://www.bpsweb.org/About.BPS/About.BPS.shtml, September 5, 2006.

6. Bertin RJ. Added qualifications: a new dimension in pharmacy specialty certification. Washington, D.C.: Board of Pharmaceutical Specialties. Accessed at http://www.bpsweb.org/Added.Qualifications/Added.Qualifications.Article.shtml, September 5, 2006.

7. Pharmacy Technician Certification Board. Actively Certified Pharmacy Technicians nationwide as of July 31, 2006. Accessed at https://www.ptcb.org/AM/Template.cfm?Section=National_Statistics&Template=/CM/HTMLDisplay.cfm&ContentID=1938, November 11, 2006.

8. US Department of Labor Occupational Safety & Health Administration. Hazard communication: foundation of workplace chemical safety programs. Accessed at http://www.osha.gov/SLTC/hazardcommunications/index.html, September 5, 2006.

CHAPTER FOUR

Drug Classifications and Formulations

This final "basics" chapter uses an organ-system approach to describe the chief actions of medications on the human body. It introduces anatomy, physiology, diseases, pathophysiology, and epidemiology and presents the most common prescription and nonprescription drugs in a large table. Then Chapter 4 briefly describes the most common formulations for drugs and presents routes of administration of drugs.

Introduction

We arrive at the topic that is at the heart of pharmacy practice: the medications them-selves. Medications are powerful substances that can have profound—even lethal (produc-ing death)—effects on the human body. In this chapter, we begin to appreciate how drugs work, what diseases can be prevented or treated with common agents, what adverse effects can be expected from these drugs, and what other adverse outcomes can be expected when medication therapy goes awry.

As with most chapters in an introductory text, you will need to consult other books for detailed information on medications and their effects. This is a complicated field, one that pharmacists study every semester during their four professional years of pharmacy school. While you do not need to know many of the details that pharmacists learn, your goal as a technician should be to attain the following level of knowledge:

- Given a generic or trade name of a commonly used drug, state the other name, drug category, available dosage forms, common adverse effects (also called side effects, but side effects can be good or bad, while adverse effects are bad), common or serious drug interactions, and storage considerations (products that need to be refrigerated or kept in special containers).
- For a common disease, state nonprescription, alternative medicine, and prescription drug options used in its treatment.
- Given a patient's drug regimen, identify possible drug-related problems involving drug interactions, drugs that should not be taken together (contraindications), and common adverse effects the patient should watch for.

With these objectives in mind, let's take a look at pharmacotherapy, or the use of medications to treat human disease.

To appreciate the effects of medications on disease, you must first have some idea of how the human body works under normal circumstances.

TABLE 4-1

Common Elements Found in the Human Body

ELEMENTS (abbreviation)	ATOMIC NUMBERS (number of protons in nucleus)	MOST COMMON STABLE ATOMIC MASSES (number of of protons plus neutrons in nucleus)	MASS OF ELEMENT FOUND IN 70-KG PERSON (kg)
Hydrogen (H)	1	1	7
Carbon (C)	6	12	16
Nitrogen (N)	7	14	1.8
Oxygen (O)	8	16	43
Sodium (Na)	11	23	0.1
Phosphorus (P)	15	31	0.780
Sulfur (S)	16	32	0.14
Chlorine (Cl)	17	35 or 37	0.095
Potassium (K)	19	39	0.14
Calcium (Ca)	20	40	1
Iron (Fe)	26	56	4.2
Iodine (I)	53	127	0.02

Sources: References 1–3.

Normal Human Anatomy and Body Function

To appreciate the effects of medications on disease, you must first have some idea of how the human body works under normal circumstances. For this reason, students of pharmacy and other health care professions spend a substantial amount of time studying *human anatomy* and normal body function, or *physiology*.

Chemical and Cellular Physiology

An atom is the most basic structure of matter. It is composed of a nucleus that contains positively charged protons and uncharged neutrons and negatively charged electrons that revolve around the nucleus much like the planets travel around the sun.

Atoms are defined by the number of protons in their nuclei. For instance, as shown in Figure 4-1, carbon has 6 protons. If that atom had 7 protons, it would no longer be carbon; instead, it would be nitrogen (Table 4-1). The number of protons in the nucleus is also referred to as the atomic number.

Atoms always have the same number of electrons as protons, and this property means that atoms are neutral—that is, they have no net positive or negative charge. An element is made up of only one type of atom and cannot be further broken down by ordinary chemical means. Ninety-six percent of the body is composed of just four elements: oxygen, carbon, hydrogen, and nitrogen (Table 4-1).

In addition to an atomic number, each element has an atomic mass number, which is the sum of its protons and neutrons. For example, carbon (abbreviated as "C") has a mass number of 12, meaning that each atom in the element has a total of 12 neutrons and protons in its nucleus. While elements generally have an equal number of protons and neutrons, not all do. In fact, the presence of one or more extra neutrons can result in an unstable configuration, and this breaks down by sending out, or emitting, radioactive particles that over time, transform the atom to the more stable configuration (see Chapter 10 for more information on medications that contain radioactive elements).

A molecule is produced when two or more atoms share electrons or combine with each other through a type of magnetic attraction. For example, a molecule of water is designated H_2O, meaning that two atoms of hydrogen (H) share electrons with one atom of oxygen (O).

Biological systems are made up largely of molecules that can be classified as sugars (carbohydrates), fats (lipids), and proteins (which often help make chemical reactions occur and are therefore called enzymes). Carbohydrates, fats, and proteins make up most of the human diet, along with vitamins and minerals such as calcium and iron.

Amino acids—20 of them—are the building blocks of proteins. Proteins can be relatively simple molecules, such as insulin, or can be very complex structures, and their effects on cells are often striking.

A cell is a living structural and functional unit surrounded by a membrane that has many substructures, as illustrated in Figure 4-2. At the center of each cell is the nucleus, which contains genetic material. As cells divide, each cell contains the same genetic material. Chromosomes are long strands of DNA, an abbreviation for deoxyribonucleic acid. In DNA, the sugar deoxyribose forms a kind of backbone in combination with phospate (phosphorus plus oxygen), and this backbone supports paired nucleotide bases composed of either thymine–cytosine or guanine–adenine. Each person has 46 chromosomes in each cell, 23 contributed from each parent.

FIGURE 4-1

Structure of a carbon atom.

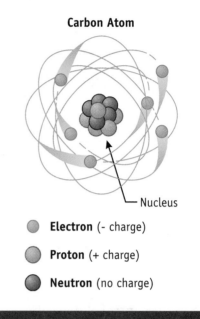

Carbon Atom

—Nucleus

● **Electron** (- charge)
● **Proton** (+ charge)
● **Neutron** (no charge)

FIGURE 4-2

Structure of the human cell (bottom), nucleus of that cell (middle), and the genetic material of the cell, DNA.

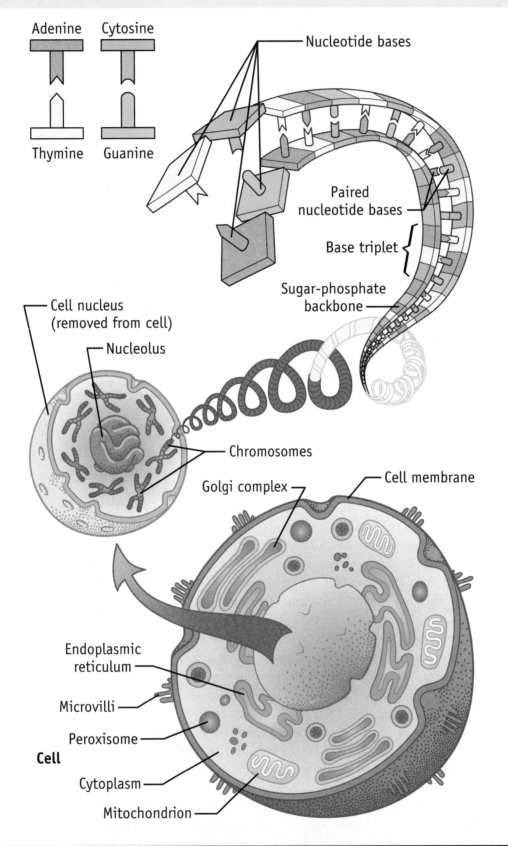

TABLE 4-2

Dosage Forms Used Commonly in Pharmaceutical Preparations

DOSAGE FORMS	DESCRIPTION	CONSIDERATIONS
SOLID ORAL DOSAGE FORMS		
Pills	Solid oral dosage forms that are made from a paste, rolled between the first finger and thumb, and then dried.	Common when pharmacists made pills in this manner in years past, but hardly any true pills are on the commercial market. Solid oral dosage forms are now tablets or capsules, and they should be referred to by these more correct names.
Tablets	Powders that are compressed with enough force that they stay together during shipping and handling but not with so much force that they will not dissolve in the body.	May be swallowed, chewed and then swallowed, dissolved under the tongue or in the buccal pouch (the space in the mouth between the teeth and the cheek), or sometimes ground up for patients who cannot swallow the whole tablet (dosage forms that contain timed-release, controlled-release, or delayed-release features should never be crushed, as it disrupts these processes).
Capsules	Gelatin containers with loose powders or timed-release beads inside. These are easily made commercially or in the pharmacy when a prescription must be compounded.	Capsules are the cheapest and easiest solid oral dosage form to make. They typically present no bioavailability problems since they dissolve easily in the fluids of the stomach and small intestine.
LIQUID DOSAGE FORMS		
Solutions	Liquids in which the drug is completely dissolved in the vehicle, making the product clear (but not necessarily colorless).	Because most drugs taste bitter, few oral solutions are used (suspensions mask the taste better). Rather, solutions are more often used for topical preparations, such as antibiotic solutions used for acne or sterile solutions that are used in the eyes.
Suspensions	A common liquid oral dosage form in which the drug is present in small particles in a flavored vehicle. Suspensions are never clear and must be shaken well to disperse the drug before a dose is measured.	Examples include liquid antibiotics used orally, anti-infective products used in the ears, and other agents prepared for pediatric or elderly patients, such as antipsychotic agents that can be given to those who will not or cannot swallow.
Syrups and elixirs	Also used to mask the bitter taste of medicines. Syrups are sweetened vehicles, while elixirs contain alcohol.	Examples include most cough syrups and elixirs such as phenobarbital.

Sections of these 46 chromosomes that code for proteins are called *genes*. Genes are characterized by the specific order and pairing of four nucleotide bases. Genes essentially code for the production of proteins within the cell, but some genes also turn on and off the activity of other genes.

Anatomy and Organ Systems

As you may remember from biology or health courses in high school, the human body is made up of many highly specialized tissues, including bones, muscles, and nerves. Specialized cells are grouped together in organs of the body, such as the lungs or stomach. Organs that interrelate to one another in function are termed *organ systems*. The body has 11 organ systems, as outlined on the following pages.[1,4]

TABLE 4-2 (continued)

Dosage Forms Used Commonly in Pharmaceutical Preparations

DOSAGE FORMS	DESCRIPTION	CONSIDERATIONS
TOPICAL AND OTHER DOSAGE FORMS		
Creams and ointments	Semisolid preparations used to deliver drugs to the skin or mucous membranes (nose, vagina). Creams are water-based and therefore easily washed off, while ointments are fat-based and resistant to removal with water.	Examples include hydrocortisone cream and ointment; contraceptive creams are used vaginally, including Ortho-Creme and Koromex.
Lotions (also called emulsions)	Lotions, products used to soften or deliver drugs to the skin, are liquid preparations that contain two "phases." Similar to how drugs can be dissolved in a solution, a water phase can be dispersed in a fat (lipid) phase in an emulsion, or small lipid globules can be dispersed in a water phase.	Examples include Calamine lotion, and the many lotions such as Curel and Vaseline Intensive Care that are used to rehydrate or soften the skin.
Transdermal patches and subdermal inserts	Drugs can be delivered through the skin using patches that control the rate of drug administration and through the use of inserts that are surgically implanted under the skin.	Examples include Nitroderm patches and Implanon contraceptive inserts.
VAGINAL, URETHRAL, AND RECTAL DOSAGE FORMS		
Suppositories	Dosage forms designed to remain solid at room or refrigerator temperature and to melt, thereby releasing the drug, when inserted into an orifice (or opening) of the body. The two most commonly used suppositories are inserted into the rectum or vagina, and a few suppositories are used in the urethra of men.	Numerous agents are formulated as rectal suppositories, including Phenergan, which is used when patients' nausea and vomiting are so severe that they cannot keep down the oral form of this drug. Vaginal suppositories include contraceptive products such as Encare and antifungal agents such as Monistat. Other vaginal contraceptives are marketed as gels, foams, and jellies.
INJECTABLE DOSAGE FORMS		
Injectable solutions	Most injectable drugs are formulated as sterile solutions. Depending on the specific drug in the solution, these can be injected into arteries, veins, or tissues or can be used to make large-volume solutions that are then infused into the body through a vein, artery, or the peritoneal cavity (the space around the stomach, intestines, liver, and other nearby organs).	Because of the high concentrations of drugs in most injectable products, be extremely careful that you use the right drug and strength. Also, some drugs cannot be given intravenously, while others cannot be injected into the muscle, for various reasons.
Injectable suspensions	A few injectable products are formulated as suspensions. These are always injected in muscle, where they are absorbed into the blood. Suspensions should never be injected into veins or arteries, since the particles in them can get stuck in the lungs and capillaries, causing serious injury or death.	Most injectable suspensions are antibiotics; these are absorbed from intramuscular injections fairly quickly. Other products, including antipsychotic agents, are made to be absorbed over a 3- or 4-week period. Since patients with schizophrenia and other psychoses are often afraid to take their medicines (they think the doctors are trying to kill them), these "depot" injections provide a way to give these patients their needed medications.
Injectable emulsions	When patients are unable to take food by mouth, they must be fed through the veins and arteries ("parenterally"). Lipid emulsions are to provide the fat that people normally get from their diets.	Examples include Liposyn, Intralipid, and Nutrilipid.

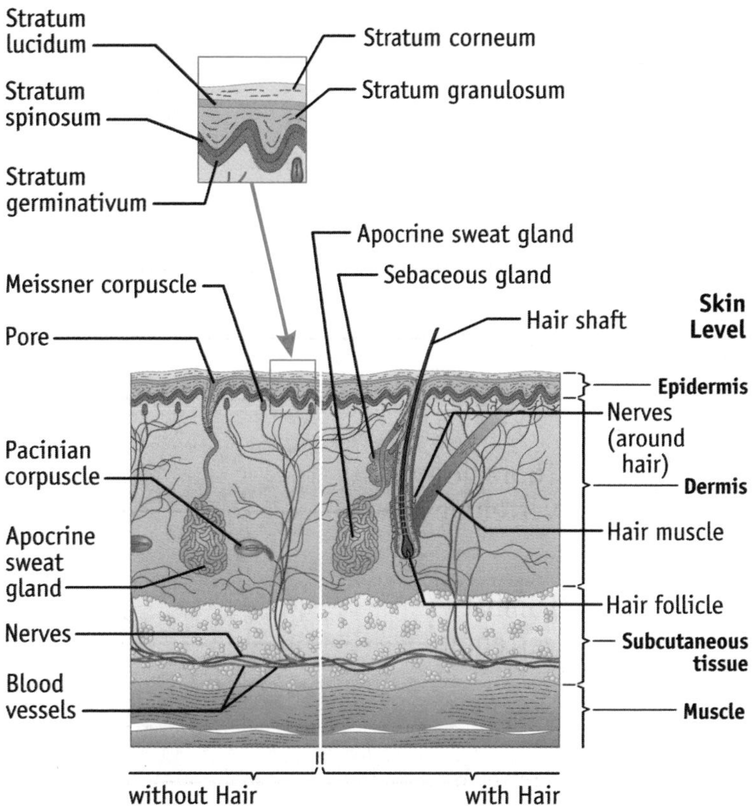

Many diseases result from disruptions in one or more of these organ systems. Drugs and drug products that are primarily used to treat these diseases are often grouped together, and you should be able to name several agents useful in treating the most common diseases affecting people. The organ system approach is generally used for making these categorizations, as shown in Table 4-4.

INTEGUMENTARY SYSTEM

The integumentary system literally holds the body together and helps it stay cool and interact with its environment. This systems includes the skin, hair, nails, and sweat glands (Figure 4-3) and is responsible for protection, body temperature regulation, conservation of water, and production of vitamin D precursors. The skin is composed of a thin, outermost area called the epidermis, under which lies the thicker dermis. Just beneath the skin is the subcutaneous tissue, which contains fat cells, blood vessels, and

FIGURE 4-3

Structure of the skin.

nerves to supply the skin. Sebaceous glands are usually connected to hair follicles and secrete an oily substance called sebum which keeps the skin and hair from drying out. Sweat glands produce around 600 mL of sweat per day, which serves to cool the body as it evaporates. Vitamin D, needed for the absorption of calcium, is made when sunlight activates a precursor located in the skin. The skin is the site of administration for many drugs, those injected into the subcutaneous tissue and those administered by transdermal patch. In both cases, in general, the drug reaches the blood and is carried throughout the body.

SKELETAL SYSTEM

The skeletal system consists of bones, cartilage, and joints (Figure 4-4). Without the skeletal system, people would be like jellyfish—incapable of initiating movement or picking up items we find in the places we live.

Adults have 206 bones, including 106 just in the hands and feet! Bones provide protection of internal organs, allow body movement, and provide attachment for skeletal muscle.

Bones are richly supplied with blood vessels and nerves. The bone marrow, located in the ends of long bones in the arms and legs and in the pelvis, ribs, sternum (breastbone), and skull, produces blood cells. Bone also stores calcium, phosphorus, and triglycerides.

Joints—formed when two bones meet—allow movement. They contain synovial fluid that lubricates the joint.

Cartilage is similar in function to bone but very different in many other ways. Cartilage, which you can feel in your ears and nose, consists of collagen fibers and does not contain blood vessels or nerves. It provides support but allows flexibility.

FIGURE 4-4

Skeletal system of the human body.

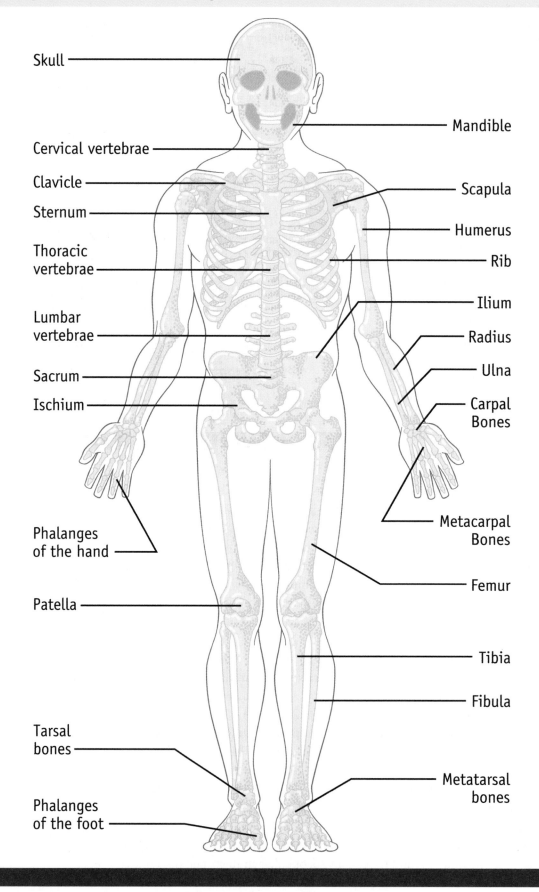

FIGURE 4-5

Front views of the muscular system of the human body.

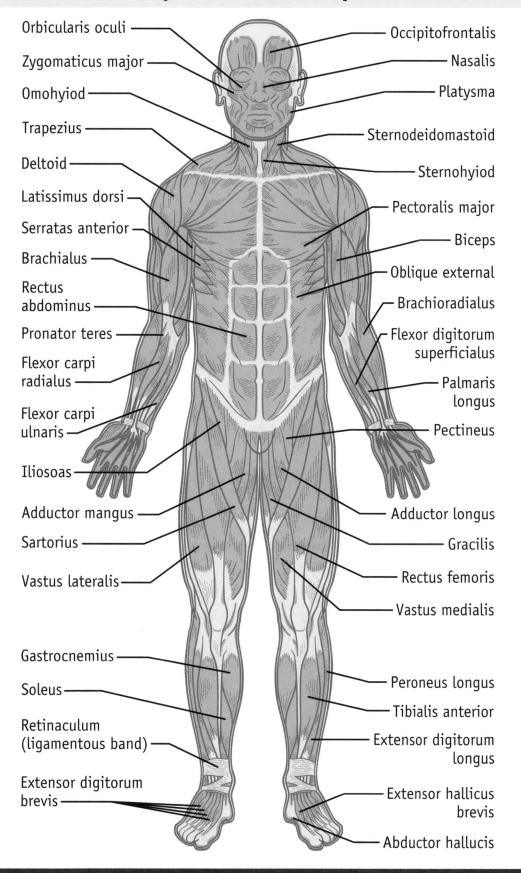

Orbicularis oculi
Zygomaticus major
Omohyiod
Trapezius
Deltoid
Latissimus dorsi
Serratas anterior
Brachialus
Rectus abdominus
Pronator teres
Flexor carpi radialus
Flexor carpi ulnaris
Iliosoas
Adductor mangus
Sartorius
Vastus lateralis
Gastrocnemius
Soleus
Retinaculum (ligamentous band)
Extensor digitorum brevis

Occipitofrontalis
Nasalis
Platysma
Sternodeidomastoid
Sternohyiod
Pectoralis major
Biceps
Oblique external
Brachioradialus
Flexor digitorum superficialus
Palmaris longus
Pectineus
Adductor longus
Gracilis
Rectus femoris
Vastus medialis
Peroneus longus
Tibialis anterior
Extensor digitorum longus
Extensor hallicus brevis
Abductor hallucis

FIGURE 4-5 (continued)

Rear view of the muscular system of the human body.

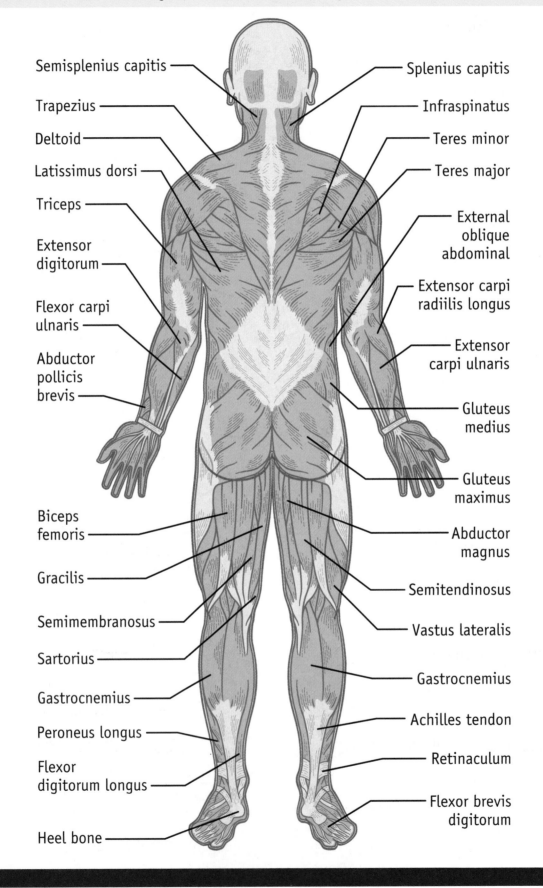

- Semisplenius capitis
- Trapezius
- Deltoid
- Latissimus dorsi
- Triceps
- Extensor digitorum
- Flexor carpi ulnaris
- Abductor pollicis brevis
- Biceps femoris
- Gracilis
- Semimembranosus
- Sartorius
- Gastrocnemius
- Peroneus longus
- Flexor digitorum longus
- Heel bone

- Splenius capitis
- Infraspinatus
- Teres minor
- Teres major
- External oblique abdominal
- Extensor carpi radiilis longus
- Extensor carpi ulnaris
- Gluteus medius
- Gluteus maximus
- Abductor magnus
- Semitendinosus
- Vastus lateralis
- Gastrocnemius
- Achilles tendon
- Retinaculum
- Flexor brevis digitorum

Normal Human Anatomy and Body Function

To appreciate the effects of medications on disease, you must first have some idea of how the human body works under normal circumstances. For this reason, students of pharmacy and other health care professions spend a substantial amount of time studying *human anatomy* and normal body function, or *physiology*.

Chemical and Cellular Physiology

An atom is the most basic structure of matter. It is composed of a nucleus that contains positively charged protons and uncharged neutrons and negatively charged electrons that revolve around the nucleus much like the planets travel around the sun.

Atoms are defined by the number of protons in their nuclei. For instance, as shown in Figure 4-1, carbon has 6 protons. If that atom had 7 protons, it would no longer be carbon; instead, it would be nitrogen (Table 4-1). The number of protons in the nucleus is also referred to as the atomic number.

Atoms always have the same number of electrons as protons, and this property means that atoms are neutral—that is, they have no net positive or negative charge. An element is made up of only one type of atom and cannot be further broken down by ordinary chemical means. Ninety-six percent of the body is composed of just four elements: oxygen, carbon, hydrogen, and nitrogen (Table 4-1).

In addition to an atomic number, each element has an atomic mass number, which is the sum of its protons and neutrons. For example, carbon (abbreviated as "C") has a mass number of 12, meaning that each atom in the element has a total of 12 neutrons and protons in its nucleus. While elements generally have an equal number of protons and neutrons, not all do. In fact, the presence of one or more extra neutrons can result in an unstable configuration, and this breaks down by sending out, or emitting, radioactive particles that over time, transform the atom to the more stable configuration (see Chapter 10 for more information on medications that contain radioactive elements).

A molecule is produced when two or more atoms share electrons or combine with each other through a type of magnetic attraction. For example, a molecule of water is designated H_2O, meaning that two atoms of hydrogen (H) share electrons with one atom of oxygen (O).

Biological systems are made up largely of molecules that can be classified as sugars (carbohydrates), fats (lipids), and proteins (which often help make chemical reactions occur and are therefore called enzymes). Carbohydrates, fats, and proteins make up most of the human diet, along with vitamins and minerals such as calcium and iron.

Amino acids—20 of them—are the building blocks of proteins. Proteins can be relatively simple molecules, such as insulin, or can be very complex structures, and their effects on cells are often striking.

A cell is a living structural and functional unit surrounded by a membrane that has many substructures, as illustrated in Figure 4-2. At the center of each cell is the nucleus, which contains genetic material. As cells divide, each cell contains the same genetic material. Chromosomes are long strands of DNA, an abbreviation for deoxyribonucleic acid. In DNA, the sugar deoxyribose forms a kind of backbone in combination with phospate (phosphorus plus oxygen), and this backbone supports paired nucleotide bases composed of either adenine–thymine or cytosine–guanine. Each person has 46 chromosomes in each cell, 23 contributed from each parent.

FIGURE 4-1

Structure of a carbon atom.

Carbon Atom

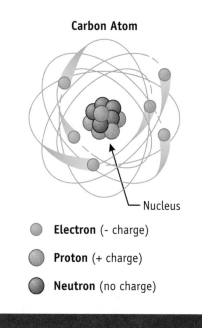

Nucleus

● **Electron** (- charge)

● **Proton** (+ charge)

● **Neutron** (no charge)

FIGURE 4-7

The five senses.

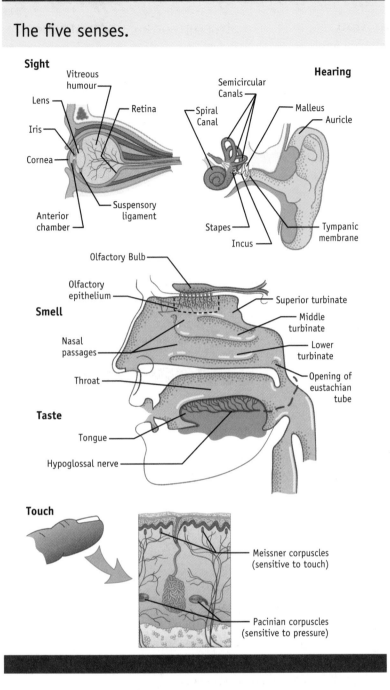

Sight

Vitreous humour
Lens
Iris
Cornea
Retina
Suspensory ligament
Anterior chamber

Hearing

Semicircular Canals
Spiral Canal
Malleus
Auricle
Stapes
Incus
Tympanic membrane

Smell

Olfactory Bulb
Olfactory epithelium
Superior turbinate
Middle turbinate
Nasal passages
Lower turbinate
Throat
Opening of eustachian tube

Taste

Tongue
Hypoglossal nerve

Touch

Meissner corpuscles (sensitive to touch)
Pacinian corpuscles (sensitive to pressure)

MUSCULAR SYSTEM

Muscles attach to bones and produce body movements, maintain posture, produce body heat, and control outflow of certain liquids (Figure 4-5). Without the muscles and associated tissues (ligaments and tendons), the body would collapse like a puppet that no one is controlling.

Three types of muscles are found in the human body:

- **Skeletal muscle** — connects to and moves bones. Impulses from nerves allow voluntary movement. Since the nerve and muscle don't directly touch, a chemical called a neurotransmitter (acetylcholine, specifically) is released from a nerve ending at the junction of the nerve and muscle to direct muscle movement.
- **Cardiac muscle** — contained in the walls of the heart and causes the heart to contract (beat). Unlike skeletal muscle, contraction is not dependant on neurotransmitters and is auto-regulated.
- **Smooth muscle** — found in blood vessels, airways, the iris of the eye, and in other hollow organs such as the bladder. Like cardiac muscle, it is not voluntarily controlled.

NERVOUS SYSTEM

The nervous system, depicted in Figure 4-6, is responsible for gathering information from in and around the body, whether it be a pin prick on the skin or a noise heard or the acidity of the blood, processing this information in the brain and determining how to react, and lastly, conveying the brain's "decision" back to the muscles, glands, and organs responsible for performing the function. In addition, nerves go to the internal organs of the body to monitor and in some cases direct activity.

Nerves that send information to the brain are called afferent nerves, and those that send information from the brain to the tissue are called efferent nerves. The nervous system is composed of the central nervous system (CNS), the brain (including the cerebellum as shown in Figure 4-6) and spinal cord, and the peripheral nervous system (PNS), all of the nerves outside of the CNS. The PNS can be further subdivided as follows:

- **Somatic nervous system** — afferent nerves gather information from the five senses (sight, smell, touch, taste, and sound, depicted in Figure 4-7) and efferent nerves return information to skeletal muscles. This system is under voluntary control.

- **Autonomic nervous system** — afferent nerves gather information from various organs such as the stomach and lungs. Efferent nerves are classified as sympathetic and parasympathetic and generally have opposing actions, like increasing versus decreasing the heart rate. This system is generally involuntary; that is, it operates without the person being aware of or in control of its actions.

ENDOCRINE SYSTEM

This system includes glands that secrete hormones and related substances that control functions such as metabolism, reproduction, and growth. Hormones are excreted in response to signals originating in the "master" glands, the hypothalamus, a part of the brain, and pituitary glands, located at the base of the brain and connected to the hypothalamus (Figure 4-8).

For example, if blood glucose (sugar) levels are low, the hypothalamus will excrete a hormone to tell the pituitary to secrete a second hormone that tells the pancreas to secrete glucagon and the liver to produce glucose. If blood glucose becomes too high, the hypothalamus secretes an inhibiting hormone that ultimately stops the production of glucose and causes the release of insulin from the pancreas. Thus, hormones are excreted via a chemical feedback mechanism.

The pineal gland, in the brain, secretes melatonin, which induces sleep. Melatonin is sold in pharmacies and other retail outlets as a dietary supplement that helps people get to sleep.

Other glands in the human body include:

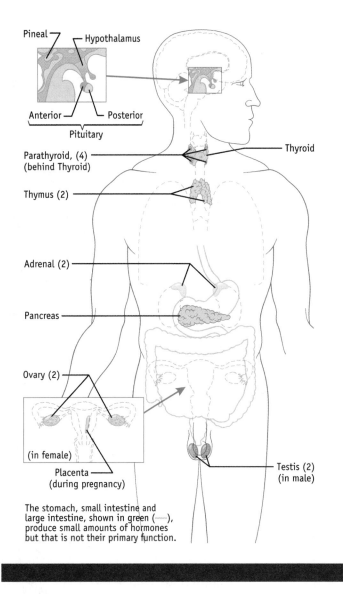

FIGURE 4-8

Endocrine system of the human body.

Pineal — Hypothalamus
Anterior — Posterior
Pituitary
Parathyroid, (4) (behind Thyroid) — Thyroid
Thymus (2)
Adrenal (2)
Pancreas
Ovary (2)
(in female)
Placenta (during pregnancy)
Testis (2) (in male)

The stomach, small intestine and large intestine, shown in green (—), produce small amounts of hormones but that is not their primary function.

- **Thyroid gland** — produces thyroid hormone, which controls cellular metabolism and regulates body temperature.
- **Parathyroid gland** — regulates body levels of calcium, phosphate, and magnesium.
- **Thymus gland** — produces hormones that promote immunity (the body's defense system against infection).
- **Adrenal glands** — produce glucocorticoids (cortisol), mineralocorticoids (aldosterone), small amounts of androgens, and epinephrine and norepinephrine. Glucocorticoids regulate metabolism and resistance to stress and have anti-inflammatory effects. Mineralocorticoids regulate blood pressure by affecting the amount of fluid retained in the circulation. Epinephrine and norepinephrine, also known as adrenaline and noradrenaline, respectively, are excreted during exercise or in stressful situations to increase heart rate and blood flow to various organs and to dilate the airways.
- **Pancreas** — secretes insulin, which lowers blood sugar (glucose) levels, and glucagon, which raises blood glucose levels.

FIGURE 4-9

Cardiovascular system of the human body.

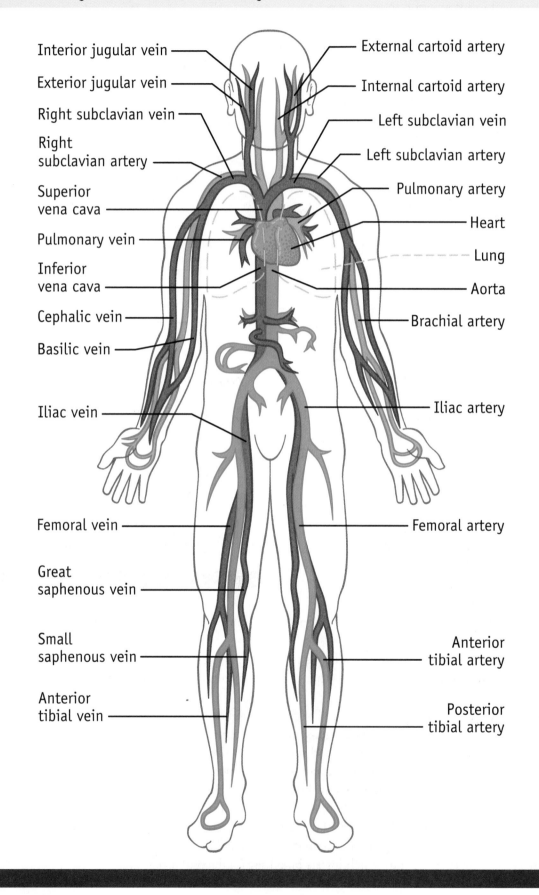

Interior jugular vein

Exterior jugular vein

Right subclavian vein

Right subclavian artery

Superior vena cava

Pulmonary vein

Inferior vena cava

Cephalic vein

Basilic vein

Iliac vein

Femoral vein

Great saphenous vein

Small saphenous vein

Anterior tibial vein

External cartoid artery

Internal cartoid artery

Left subclavian vein

Left subclavian artery

Pulmonary artery

Heart

Lung

Aorta

Brachial artery

Iliac artery

Femoral artery

Anterior tibial artery

Posterior tibial artery

FIGURE 4-9

60   DRUG CLASSIFICATIONS AND FORMULATIONS

FIGURE 4-10

Lymphatic system of the human body.

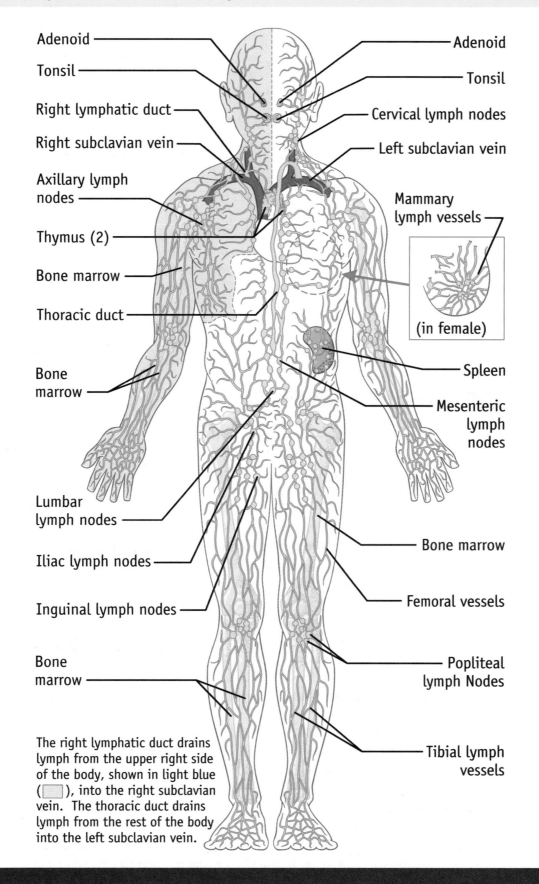

Adenoid

Tonsil

Right lymphatic duct

Right subclavian vein

Axillary lymph nodes

Thymus (2)

Bone marrow

Thoracic duct

Bone marrow

Lumbar lymph nodes

Iliac lymph nodes

Inguinal lymph nodes

Bone marrow

Adenoid

Tonsil

Cervical lymph nodes

Left subclavian vein

Mammary lymph vessels

(in female)

Spleen

Mesenteric lymph nodes

Bone marrow

Femoral vessels

Popliteal lymph Nodes

Tibial lymph vessels

The right lymphatic duct drains lymph from the upper right side of the body, shown in light blue ( ), into the right subclavian vein. The thoracic duct drains lymph from the rest of the body into the left subclavian vein.

FIGURE 4-11

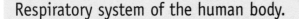

Respiratory system of the human body.

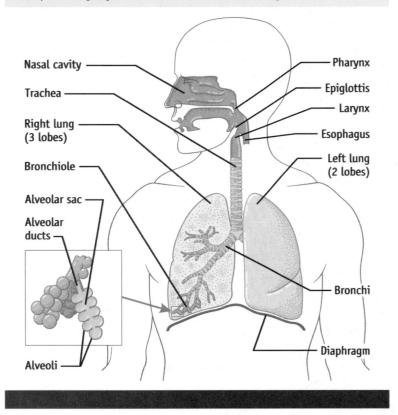

Nasal cavity

Trachea

Right lung
(3 lobes)

Bronchiole

Alveolar sac

Alveolar
ducts

Alveoli

Pharynx

Epiglottis

Larynx

Esophagus

Left lung
(2 lobes)

Bronchi

Diaphragm

- **Ovaries (in girls and women)** — produce estrogen and progesterone, which regulate the menstrual cycle, maintain pregnancy and lactation, and promote development of female sexual characteristics.
- **Testes (in boys and men)** — produces testosterone, needed for sperm production and male sexual characteristics.

CARDIOVASCULAR SYSTEM

The cardiovascular system consists of the heart, blood vessels, and blood (Figure 4-9). It is responsible for transporting nutrients, waste products, gases, and hormones; some immune functions; and regulation of temperature. This system has many parts, including the following:

- **Heart** — The heart contains four chambers and four valves. The right atrium receives blood from the body through the superior and inferior vena cava. It is then pumped through the tricuspid valve into the right ventricle, which pumps blood to the lungs through the pulmonary valve into the right and left pulmonary arteries.

From the lungs, oxygenated blood is received back into the heart through the pulmonary veins, into the left atrium. Blood passes through the bicuspid valve into the left ventricle. The left ventricle pumps blood throughout the body through the aortic valve and into the aorta.

- **Blood vessels** — Blood vessels that carry blood from the heart are called arteries. Arterial blood contains oxygen (except for the blood in the pulmonary arteries, which carry oxygen from the right side of the heart to the lungs where oxygenation occurs). Capillaries are very small blood vessels that connect arteries and veins, and this is where nutrients and gases are exchanged within the tissues. Veins carry blood back to the heart. Since the oxygen has been released into the tissues, venous blood is deoxygenated (except for blood within the pulmonary veins, which go from the lungs to the left side of the heart for pumping to the tissues). The heart muscle itself is also fed by coronary arteries and veins.
- **Blood** — Blood contains a liquid portion called plasma. Plasma is mostly water but also contains proteins and other solutes. Plasma without the clotting proteins is called serum. In addition to plasma, blood contains many cells, including red blood cells (erythrocytes), which carry oxygen; white blood cells (leukocytes), which are of many types but generally fight infections and aid in immune responses; and platelets (thrombocytes), which aid in blood clotting.

LYMPHATIC SYSTEM

The lymphatic system is made up of lymphatic tissue, lymphatic vessels, and lymph fluid (Figure 4-10). This system is key in fighting infection and maintaining immune response to foreign substances. It also plays a role in draining excess fluid and transporting fat.

Cells important in providing an immune response to a foreign substance, T cells and B cells, are produced in lymphatic tissue, which includes the bone marrow, thymus gland, lymph nodes, spleen, adenoids, and tonsils.

Lymph is a clear fluid that bathes cells. It flows through lymphatic vessels into the subclavian vein to rid the body of excess fluid.

RESPIRATORY SYSTEM

The respiratory system includes the nasal cavity, pharynx (throat), larynx (voice box), trachea (windpipe), bronchi, and lungs (Figure 4-11). The primary function of this system is the exchange of gases that occurs between the alveoli and the capillaries.

Oxygen (O_2) is absorbed here into the blood from the air that has been breathed in. Carbon dioxide (CO_2), a byproduct of cellular metabolism, is released from the blood and exhaled through the respiratory system. If CO_2 builds up, the blood becomes too acidic (that is, the pH, or hydrogen ion content of the blood, is too low), and this is toxic to cells. Similarly, if the pH of the blood is too high, the blood becomes too basic, and this too can damage cells throughout the body. Thus, the respiratory system is essential to maintaining the right concentration of hydrogen ions in the body. This is referred to as acid–base balance.

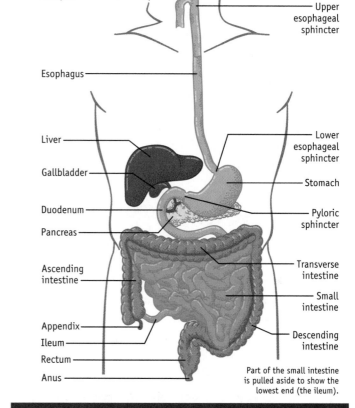

FIGURE 4-12

Gastrointestinal system of the human body.

Pharynx

Upper esophageal sphincter

Esophagus

Liver

Lower esophageal sphincter

Gallbladder

Stomach

Duodenum

Pyloric sphincter

Pancreas

Ascending intestine

Transverse intestine

Small intestine

Appendix

Ileum

Descending intestine

Rectum

Anus

Part of the small intestine is pulled aside to show the lowest end (the ileum).

The respiratory system also permits the sense of smell, filters air that is breathed in, and produces sound (voice) as exhaled air interacts with the larynx in the throat.

DIGESTIVE SYSTEM

The digestive, or gastroenterologic, system consists of the gastrointestinal tract, which runs from the mouth to the anus, and accessory digestive organs such as the pancreas, gallbladder, and liver (Figure 4-12). These structures have the following functions:

- **Gastrointestinal tract** — comprises the pharynx, esophagus, stomach, small intestine (duodenum, jejunum, and ileum), large intestine or colon, and rectum. Its job is to process food from the time it is eaten until it is digested, or broken down into small subunits, and then absorbed or eliminated. The degree of acidity changes along the gastrointestinal tract, and this affects the absorption and breakdown of food and drugs. In the stomach, the pH is low (very acidic), causing ingested substances to be broken down, but little absorption occurs for most nutrients and drugs. One notable exception is ethanol—the alcohol people consume in beverages—which is absorbed from the stomach, and this accounts for its rapid onset of effects. Nutrients, water, and drugs are primarily absorbed in the small intestine, where the pH is higher (more basic).

FIGURE 4-13

Drug metabolism in the liver.

Medications absorbed from the small intestines generally are taken directly to the liver, where some are not metabolized at all, others are metabolized to a small degree (top diagram), and others are metabolized to a great degree (bottom diagram).

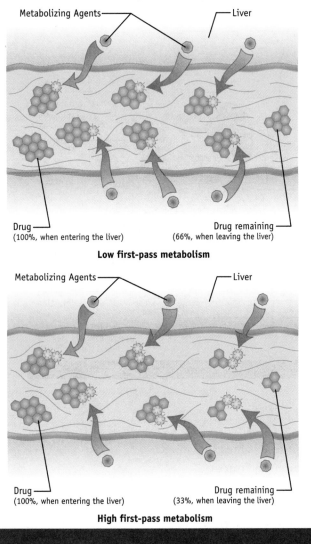

Metabolizing Agents — Liver

Drug
(100%, when entering the liver)

Drug remaining
(66%, when leaving the liver)

Low first-pass metabolism

Metabolizing Agents — Liver

Drug
(100%, when entering the liver)

Drug remaining
(33%, when leaving the liver)

High first-pass metabolism

- **Pancreas** — produces and secretes pancreatic enzymes that aid in breaking down food. The pancreas also produces hormones such as insulin and glucagon. These were mentioned above under the discussion of the endocrine system, and they are important in patients who have diabetes.

- **Liver** — detoxifies or breaks down ingested substances. The liver secretes bile, which is needed for fat absorption and is important in the breakdown or metabolism of carbohydrates and proteins. It also helps in maintaining the proper blood glucose level, stores some vitamins and minerals, and produces compounds that allow the blood to clot when needed. As shown in Figure 4-13, drugs are often metabolized (broken down or inactivated) in the liver by various hepatic (liver) enzymes (specialized proteins that facilitate chemical changes), the cytochrome P450 enzymes, and these are involved in many drug interactions when two drugs are metabolized by the same enzyme, or when one drug alters the function of an enzyme responsible for metabolizing a second drug. Also, drugs absorbed from the intestines are carried directly to the liver, where they undergo first-pass metabolism. As shown in the lower part of Figure 4-13, some drugs are extensively metabolized at this point, meaning that only a small part of an oral dose actually reaches the general circulation of the body. This is called high, or extensive, first-pass metabolism. Drugs that undergo little transformation are said to undergo low first-pass metabolism. Metabolism is discussed further later in this chapter in the section on Pharmacokinetics.

- **Gallbladder** — stores bile, a yellowish-green substance that when secreted through bile ducts into the small intestine, helps the body emulsify fats so that they can be absorbed into the blood.

URINARY SYSTEM

The urinary system consists of two kidneys, two ureters, a bladder, and a urethra (Figure 4-14). The kidneys filter blood and remove unnecessary substances and excess water. Regulation of electrolyte levels (e.g., sodium, potassium, calcium, chloride) is maintained by the kidneys. The kidneys help maintain acid–base balance (which is also regulated by the respiratory system, as described above) by regulating the amount of hydrogen ions and bicarbonate ions that are excreted.

The kidneys also control blood pressure by regulating the amount of water excreted and also by releasing enzymes that constrict or dilate the blood vessels. Urine produced by the kidneys is transported through the ureters to the bladder, a storage container, until released through the urethra, which terminates in the penis in men and boys and at the vaginal opening in girls and women. In men, the urethra travels through a doughnut-shaped organ, the prostate gland, and men with benign prostatic hypertrophy, or BPH, have problems with urination because of the inflammation associated with BPH.

FIGURE 4-14

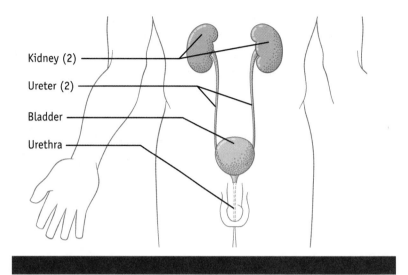

Urinary system of the human body.

Kidney (2)
Ureter (2)
Bladder
Urethra

REPRODUCTIVE SYSTEM

The male and female reproductive systems, depicted in Figure 4-15, are responsible for propagation of the human species, that is, making babies. Men produce sperm, and these, when united with an egg from the woman, form a zygote. The zygote implants in the lining of the uterus, where it develops into a fetus and then a baby, which is normally delivered 36–40 weeks later.

Female reproductive organs are as follows:
- **Ovaries** — produce and release eggs and hormones (estrogen and progesterone)
- **Fallopian tubes** — connect the ovaries to the uterus and are the site of fertilization
- **Uterus** — where a fertilized egg implants to grow into a fetus
- **Vagina** — a passageway for sperm and menstrual flow, and childbirth
- **Vulva** — collective term for external female genitals
- **Mammary tissue (breasts)** — produce milk for infants

Male reproductive organs include these structures:
- **Testes** — produce sperm and secrete the hormone testosterone
- **Scrotum** — a sac containing the testes
- **Prostate gland** — helps produce semen
- **Penis** — contains the urethra and is a passageway for semen and urine

Physiology: Body Function

If anatomy provides a picture of the human body, physiology is a movie. In other words, anatomy describes the body at rest, but the living body is never at rest. The heart is beating, blood is moving through veins and arteries, sensory nerves are detecting changes in the environment, brain cells are interpreting input and returning instructions, the intestines are processing nutrients, and the kidneys are eliminating wastes. The study of the ways in which the body and its organ systems work is *physiology*.

Just as drugs can be described as affecting certain organs or organ systems, the actions of many agents are known to be specific to the physiologic processes of one or more organs. Because our knowledge of medical science is so much more complete than in the past (and rapidly increasing each year), medications have been developed that target cell defects and disrupted physiologic processes more specifically. These medicines then work more effectively and with fewer adverse effects than many older drugs.

FIGURE 4-15

Male and female reproductive systems of the human body.

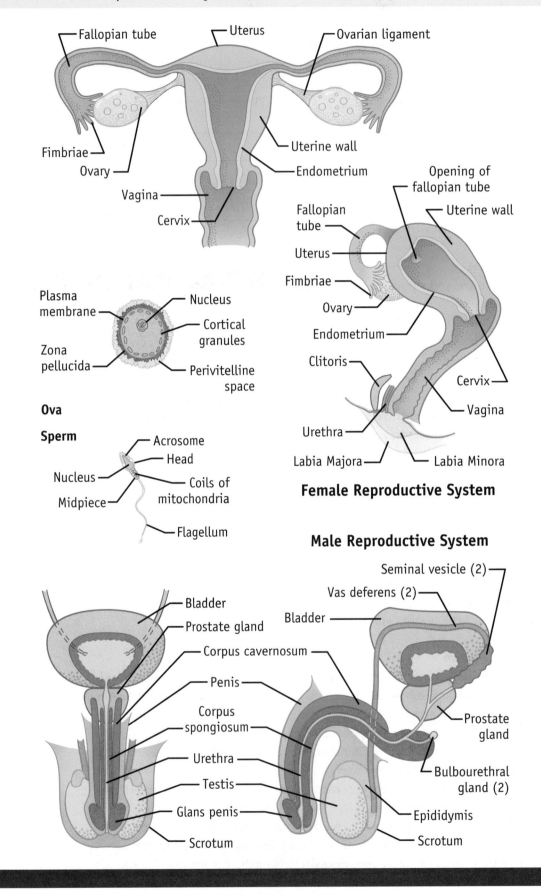

Female Reproductive System

Male Reproductive System

Pathophysiology: When Something Is Wrong

When the body is working as it normally does, a state of *homeostasis* is said to exist. The body is able to perform all the functions expected of it, the organs and organ systems are working in concert with each other, nutrients and oxygen are being distributed to cells throughout the body, and wastes are being processed and eliminated by the lungs, kidneys, and intestines.

When something disrupts this homeostasis, an abnormal state ensues—one we call *disease*. Some diseases cause or are the result of problems at the cell level, including adaptation, injury, growth, or death. This disruption may be caused by many different factors:

- Poisons or harmful substances that have entered the body
- Microorganisms such as bacteria, viruses, or fungi
- Lack of nutrients or oxygen
- A breakdown in the body's response to microorganisms or other foreign matter
- Products of genes that occur in some (but not all) people
- Aging of the body
- Unknown factors

The study of what goes wrong in diseases is called *pathophysiology*. By understanding the pathophysiology of diseases and knowing what drugs are available that affect those abnormal processes, you can readily understand which drugs are used for which diseases.

Before a drug is used to treat a disease, the physician or other prescriber must be sure that the patient has the suspected disease. This occurs through the process of *diagnosis*. In making a diagnosis, the physician considers the patient and his or her race, age, sex, family and medical histories, and genetic makeup; how the patient feels; the results of the physical examination and laboratory tests; and therapies that have worked in other people with similar clinical presentations. With this knowledge, the physician can (generally) make a definitive diagnosis and outline a reasonable treatment plan that will provide the best chance of compensating for or correcting the disease.

Pharmacists do not usually make diagnoses, as their expertise lies more in knowing about treatments. However, patients routinely ask pharmacists for assistance with nonprescription drugs and dietary supplements, all sold without a prescription, and this can involve determining what is causing the bothersome symptoms. In addition, as discussed in the chapter on Governance, a third category of drug products is emerging, one consisting of medications that are kept behind the pharmacy counter. If this trend continues, pharmacists may need to do more assessment of patient problems than has been common in the past.

Risk Factors for Disease

Simply put, *risk factors* are those characteristics unique to a given patient that increase his or her odds of having a particular disease. Examples of the relationships between disease and risk factors include the following:

- Hypertension is more common among blacks than whites, and it tends to occur in families, indicating a *genetic predisposition*.
- Depression is more common among women than men, and depression and suicide are more likely to occur in a patient when one or more first-degree relatives (father, mother, brother, sister) also have had depression or attempted or committed suicide.
- Diabetes is more common among blacks, Hispanics, American Indians, and Asian Americans, and *sedentary lifestyles* (not getting much exercise) increase the risk of diabetes, especially type 2 diabetes (formerly referred to as non-insulin-dependent diabetes).

- For many diseases, including type 2 diabetes and Alzheimer's disease, older patients are at greater risk than are younger patients.

Thus, risk factors are an important part of the clinical evaluation of patients and provide valuable evidence for reaching a decision about diagnosis. In addition, patients should be aware of their own risk factors so that they can make appropriate adjustments in their lifestyle. For instance, improving diet, getting more exercise, and reducing or eliminating the use of tobacco and alcohol can decrease the risk of getting certain diseases.

An area of increasing importance to genetic risk factors in the early 21st century is gene therapy and pharmacogenomics. The Human Genome Project, an effort supported by the National Institutes of Health, has mapped the location of every human gene on the 23 chromosome pairs. Pharmaceutical companies are starting to use this information to produce therapies that may be able to correct serious genetic defects before people are born or when they are very young. People may also be able to learn early in their lives which diseases are likely to cause them problems later in life. They can then use this information to reduce their risks of getting the disease. For instance, if someone knows he or she has a genetic predisposition to high cholesterol, special diets, monitoring, and perhaps drug therapy could begin early in life before damage occurs to the arteries and other structures of the body. It will be interesting and exciting to see what new frontiers gene therapy and genomics open up for medical science and pharmacotherapy.

Signs and Symptoms of Disease

In addition to risk factors, two other types of evidence help the clinician reach a diagnosis:

- Subjective clues, or how the patient describes the condition, are referred to as *signs* of the disease.
- Objective clues, or what the physician or other health professionals find during physical examination and laboratory or other tests, are called *symptoms* of the disease.

Working the clues through a diagnostic framework, the physician rules out various possibilities until one or more diseases remain. At times, physicians cannot determine for sure which disease is present and must try therapy for one of the possibilities empirically (without knowing for sure) to see whether the patient's condition improves. If it does, then that disease is assumed to be present; if it does not, therapy can then be tried for a second possibility, and so on, until the correct diagnosis is determined.

Epidemiology: Studying Large Numbers of People

Epidemiology provides valuable knowledge by analyzing populations of people, rather than just individuals. A good example of the application of epidemiology is when food poisoning occurs at a school or other large gathering of people. By combining information on which people with food poisoning ate which foods, the dish that caused the food poisoning can be identified. If each patient were analyzed individually, and the clues from one person were not applied to the next, investigators could never figure out which dish was the culprit.

Likewise, many important ideas about disease and pharmacotherapy have been identified based on epidemiology. Researchers have been able to figure out, for example, that a virus causes acquired immunodeficiency syndrome (AIDS), which drugs cause which adverse effects, and that high cholesterol levels are associated with heart disease.

Pharmacotherapy: Treating Disease with Drugs

After a diagnosis is made, treatment can begin. Several different options are available for treating most diseases:

- **Lifestyle modifications** — Changing the patient's diet, exercise level, or physical surroundings (for example, removing a pet from a home if the patient has asthma or is allergic to the pet)
- **Decreasing risk factors** — Eliminating tobacco, alcohol, illicit drugs, or other modifiable factors
- **Surgery** — Performing medical interventions that eliminate the cause or correct a problem
- **Pharmacotherapy** — Treating with prescription or nonprescription medications or dietary supplements such as vitamins and minerals or herbal products

Our focus in this chapter is on pharmacotherapy, especially treatment with prescription drugs. To understand what drugs do in the body, you must understand basic principles of pharmacokinetics and pharmacodynamics.

Pharmacokinetics: How Drugs Move Through the Body

Pharmacokinetics is the study of the movement of drugs through the body. Complicated mathematical models and equations are used by pharmacists to calculate doses of drugs. For some agents, the *therapeutic doses,* or doses that produce the desired effects in people, vary from person to person. Some medications may be *toxic* in some patients, even at doses that do not produce excessive effects in other people. The value of pharmacokinetics lies in the prevention of drug-related toxicity in patients by increasing the chances that the right dose will be used in each patient.

When a drug is placed into the human body, four processes describe its movement: *absorption, distribution, metabolism,* and *excretion.* By understanding the processes for each drug, pharmacists and other health professionals are able to predict doses and blood levels of drugs using pharmacokinetic equations. Let's look at each of these areas.

Absorption is the process through which the drug enters the blood. Whether injected into tissues, absorbed through the skin from a transdermal patch, inhaled into the nose or lungs, or taken by mouth, drugs must generally reach the blood to be transported to *active sites,* where they exert their therapeutic, adverse, and toxic effects. Only intravenous doses of drugs skip the process of absorption, because they are injected directly into the blood, and even then, the drugs usually move from the blood into one or more cells or tissues to exert a therapeutic effect (see below discussion of distribution).

To understand the process of absorption, suppose a 1-g dose is administered by mouth in the form of a tablet. It might break apart in the gastric juices of the stomach and pass to the small intestine in little particles. This process is called disintegration. As the pH

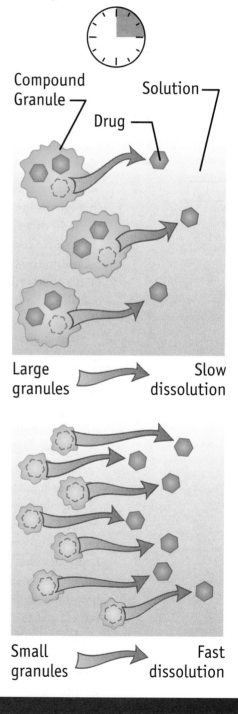

FIGURE 4-16

Dissolution: Making Drugs Available for Absorption.

Drugs administered in tablets or capsules must dissolve in gastrointestinal fluids before they can be absorbed into the body's bloodstream. The size of the particles inside a tablet or capsule can affect this rate of dissolution, as shown here.

Specific time interval

Compound Granule

Solution

Drug

Large granules → Slow dissolution

Small granules → Fast dissolution

(hydrogen ion concentration) rises in the small intestine, the drug might move from the particles and into the gastrointestinal fluids in a process called dissolution (Figure 4-16). Once a drug dissolves in the gastrointestinal fluids, it is available to be absorbed through the wall of the intestine and into the blood.

Bioavailability is the term used to describe the ratio between the amount of drug that reaches the blood and the amount of drug placed into the body. For instance, of the 1-g dose administered in the above example, only 0.9 g reaches the blood. This ratio, $\frac{0.9}{1.0}$, represents the oral bioavailability of the drug. It is usually expressed as a decimal fraction (0.9) or percentage (90%).

As mentioned under the above digestive system section, absorbed materials from the gastrointestinal tract go directly to the liver so that the body can check them for foreign or unwanted substances. The liver, the main metabolizing organ in the body, might detect this drug and convert half of it to inactive metabolites before it ever leaves the liver. This first-pass metabolism reduces the bioavailability to 45% $\left(\frac{0.9}{2 \times 100} \right)$.

Distribution is the movement of the drug through the blood and into various cells or tissues where it exerts its effect. Again, pharmacokineticists have developed various models and equations that can be used to describe this movement mathematically. The models use the concept of "compartments" to reflect the amounts of drugs in various fluids, tissues, and organs. For instance, the drug concentration might be 3 mcg/mL in the blood compartment, 3 ng/mL in the brain compartment, and 30 mcg/g in a fat tissue compartment. The high amount of drug that has distributed into fat tissue in this example means the drug would likely stay in the body for a long time because fat tissue has no way of getting rid of the drug until it moves, or partitions, back into the blood. The extent to which a drug distributes through various compartments is described mathematically as its volume of distribution. In the example of this drug that distributes into fat tissue, the drug would be said to have a large volume of distribution.

Metabolism describes the chemical changes made to the drug by the body, often by the liver but sometimes by the gastrointestinal tract wall, kidneys, lungs, or blood. As noted in the above discussion of absolute bioavailability, the liver is the main metabolizing organ of the body. It has many special proteins, called enzymes, that can change—that is, metabolize—drugs into inactive compounds, or metabolites. These enzymes are contained in special structures of the liver, the cytochrome P-450 system, which are depicted in Figure 4-13. As mentioned under the preceding discussion of the liver, many drugs interact with one another because they both have effects on or are metabolized by specific enzymes in this system. These enzymes are categorized by their function and structure and given names like 1A2 and 3C4.

Metabolism usually changes the drug from an active entity, capable of producing effects in the body, to an inactive chemical that has no effect on the body. Some drugs are metabolized into compounds that exert actions in the body (active metabolites). Other times, the body converts an inactive chemical, called a prodrug, into an active drug. Prodrugs are usually designed by pharmaceutical scientists to be absorbed or distributed better, and the body's metabolism apparatus is then used to convert the prodrug into the active drug after it has cleared this hurdle or barrier.

Excretion is the process through which the drug or its metabolites leave the body, usually in the urine or feces but sometimes through the lungs (Figure 4-17). Drugs can be excreted as either active drugs or inactive metabolites. Oftentimes, the changes made by the liver during metabolism convert the drug into a form that is easier for the kidneys or intestines to eliminate. The amount of drug excreted or metabolized to inactive compounds in a given organ or tissue over a certain amount of time is expressed mathematically as its clearance for that organ or tissue. The time it takes for the serum drug concentration to decline by one half is called the drug's half-life.

An interesting example of absorption, distribution, metabolism, and excretion is that of alcohol, one of the most commonly used—and abused—drugs in our society. Alcohol, administered in the form of a liquid, is absorbed in the stomach and the first part of the small intestine, which is why people feel the effects of alcohol so quickly when it is consumed on an empty stomach. Once absorbed, alcohol moves through the blood and into the brain, where it acts as a central nervous system depressant. That is,

FIGURE 4-17

Medications, or their metabolites, can be eliminated from the body in the urine, feces, sweat, or exhaled air.

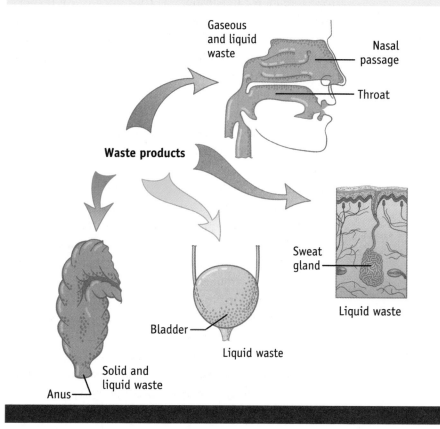

it slows down the transmission of impulses among the nerves in the brain. It does this in a dose-dependent fashion—the higher the alcohol concentration, the more effect it exerts on the brain.

Alcohol is metabolized in the liver, lungs, urine, and sweat to inactive compounds, including acetaldehyde. The amount of acetaldehyde and other metabolites produced is predictably proportional to the amount of alcohol in the blood, and a predictable amount of acetaldehyde is excreted through the lungs and into the breath (expired air). This relationship is the basis for the breath test used by police to estimate the blood alcohol concentrations in drivers of automobiles. So, as you can see, pharmacokinetics has practical applications, even outside medicine.

Pharmacodynamics: What Drugs Do in the Body

In the previous section on pharmacokinetics, most of the discussion focuses on the concentration of drug in the blood. But most drugs do not exert any effect on the blood, so that concentration is irrelevant if the drug never produces its desired effects in target tissues. The study of the relationship between serum or tissue drug levels and drug effects is called pharmacodynamics.

For most medications, a relationship between drug levels and therapeutic or toxic effects can be described mathematically using pharmacodynamics. For instance, higher concentrations of blood pressure drugs have more antihypertensive effects than do lower concentrations. In the alcohol example mentioned in the last section, the effects of alcohol can be related to the blood concentration. At low concentrations, about 50 mg/dL, a

Therapeutic doses, or doses that produce the desired effects in people, vary from person to person.

Some drugs, such as digoxin and warfarin, have doses that can be therapeutic in one patient but toxic in another.

feeling of well-being (euphoria) is produced. As the blood alcohol rises to 100 mg/dL, impairment of motor functions (speech, reaction time, balance) begins, and this worsens to severe motor impairment as the concentration rises to 150 mg/dL. Between 150 mg/dL and 250 mg/dL, nausea and dysphoria replace the earlier euphoria, and consciousness is lost at about 300 mg/dL. If the person continues to drink before passing out, then alcohol is still being absorbed from the gastrointestinal tract, and the blood alcohol level will keep rising. At about 400 mg/dL, the person will enter a coma, and if breathing stops, the person will die.

Strengths and Dosage Forms: How Drugs Are Administered

Drugs are commercially available in various strengths and dosage forms. The strength of a drug is the amount contained in a unit of the product, whether a tablet or a teaspoonful of a liquid (for example, diazepam 5-mg tablets or amoxicillin suspension 150 mg/5 mL). When preparing a prescription, you must be very careful to select the correct strength of the drug. Some drugs, such as digoxin and warfarin, have doses that can be therapeutic in one patient but toxic in another. Such medicines are said to have narrow therapeutic ranges or indexes. In the pharmacy, you may find that the various strengths of such drugs are placed on shelves away from each other; they are separated to decrease the chances of someone accidentally picking up the wrong strength.

Many drugs also come in various dosage forms. Table 4-2 defines the most common dosage forms and provides considerations about the use of each. While giving a patient the wrong dosage form may not be as serious an error as the wrong drug or strength, it can still be problematic. For instance, an elderly patient may not be able to swallow tablets or capsules and therefore may require liquid preparations. Or a patient who is vomiting may require a rectal suppository rather than oral dosage forms. Be sure you have the correct dosage form—don't assume anything!

Commonly Used Drugs and Drug Categories

Table 4-4 presents the basic facts about many of the drugs most commonly used in the United States. As you work in pharmacy, the generic and trade names of these agents will become very familiar to you. To speed this process along, you should memorize those drugs on this list that you encounter most often in your own workplace. Depending on the kind of pharmacy where you work, you may need to add to the list other drugs that are used frequently in your setting.

The column headings used in Table 4-4 and other commonly used terms deserve special mention, as shown in Table 4-3.

Drug Misadventures: When Something Goes Wrong with Pharmacotherapy

You may have seen on television or in newspapers stories about patients who died or were injured after being given the wrong drug or the wrong dose by pharmacists. Just as in the rest of life, when something can go wrong in medicine and pharmacy, it will. Despite all the training of physicians and pharmacists, even though we have the systems in place to prevent errors from happening, and although the medications are administered by intelligent patients or well-educated nurses, errors still sometimes occur.

All situations in which drugs cause unexpected harm are lumped together under terms such as *drug-related problems* (DRPs) or *drug misadventures*. These situations vary considerably, as shown in Table 4-5.

DRPs and drug misadventures are of great concern at this time. Several studies during the 1990s estimated that as many as 200,000 people die each year of DRPs in hospitals

TABLE 4-3

Description of Elements in Table 4-4

The following further explains some of the elements in Table 4-4

- **Generic name:** The generic name is the name given to each drug by the United States Adopted Names (USAN) program, a joint project of the American Medical Association, the United States Pharmacopeial Convention, and APhA. Any company that markets this drug is required by the Food and Drug Administration (FDA) to place its generic name on the package label in size at least half of that of the company's own brand name. Notice that related drugs have similar suffixes to their generic names. For instance, all the lipid-lowering agents end in –statin (for example, lovastatin, pravastatin, simvastatin). This clue will help you remember which drugs are similar.

- **Brand name:** The brand name, also called the proprietary name, is given to the product by the company marketing it. For instance, lovastatin is Mevacor, pravastatin is Pravachol, and simvastatin is Zocor. While some names relate to some fact about the drug (for instance, Premarin reflects the fact that the drug is obtained from *pregnant mare's urine*), many trade names are generated by marketing departments because people react well to them or relate them to something about the drug (for instance, the male impotence drug Viagra rhymes with Niagara, the waterfalls in upstate New York).

- **Dosage forms:** As discussed above and in Table 4-2, drugs are marketed in various dosage forms according to the intended route of administration. Oral (by mouth) is the most familiar route of administration, but this sometimes is impractical. For example, if the drug cannot be absorbed into the blood from the gastrointestinal tract or is immediately broken down after absorption (i.e., insulin) or if a person is too sick to be able to swallow a drug, then another route of administration becomes necessary. "Injectable" means only that the drug is intended for injection, which could mean into a muscle (intramuscular), vein (intravascular), skin (subcutaneous), or other tissue, so it is important to know precisely how and where the drug should be injected. Topical administration implies that the drug is absorbed into the skin. At least some of the dose may reach the circulation and produce systemic (whole body) effects.

- **Common uses:** Drugs are officially approved for treatment or prevention of certain diseases by the FDA. These uses are called the "approved indications" for that drug. However, once a drug is released onto the US market, prescribers can use it for any indication they believe is medically appropriate. When such uses become widespread or confirmed in clinical studies, these uses of the drug are listed in pharmacy reference books as "unapproved indications."

- **Adverse effects:** Drugs have both good and bad effects on the body. The adverse effects are important considerations when choosing a drug. Adverse effects, sometimes called side effects, are drug actions that occur at normal doses of a drug (in other words, when the right amount of a drug has been given). The terms toxicities and toxic effects generally refer to those effects that are produced when too much of a drug is used. Listed in the adverse effects column of Table 4-4 are the *common* and *serious* adverse effects of medications. Common adverse effects are those that many patients will encounter, and pharmacists typically warn patients about these problems and what to do if they occur. Serious adverse effects, while usually occurring rarely, are the problems that prescribers and pharmacists watch for during medication therapy.

COMMENTS, WHICH MAY INCLUDE:

- **Contraindications/Precautions:** Because of their effects on multiple organs or organ systems in the body, certain drugs either cannot be used or must be used with caution in patients with more than one disease. For instance, some of the drugs found in nonprescription cough and cold products—the decongestants—can raise blood pressure and affect blood sugar levels. Therefore, the contraindications for decongestants include patients with diseases of blood pressure or blood sugar; that is, they should not be used by patients with hypertension or diabetes. Another common contraindication is patient *allergy* to a drug. When patients allergic to one drug tend to react to other similar drugs (such as the penicillins), the drugs are said to exhibit *cross sensitivities*. Sometimes drugs can be used in patients with certain diseases, but only with caution. These warnings are listed as *precautions* to use of a drug. A common type of precaution is about the use of the drug in special patient populations, including women who are or may become pregnant, newborn babies (neonates), children, the elderly, and those with diseases of the liver (affecting metabolism) or kidneys (affecting excretion).

- **Storage considerations:** All drugs will degrade, or be changed into other substances, when exposed to oxygen and/or water, even the amounts present in the air. The rate at which drugs degrade is a function of their chemical structure and the conditions under which they are stored. Since colder temperatures slow down these degradation processes, some drugs must be frozen (below 0°C or 32°F) or stored in the refrigerator (2–8°C, or 36–46°F). Other agents can be stored at room temperature (15–30°C, or 59–86°F) but must be protected from extreme temperatures, usually high temperatures but sometimes also freezing.

TABLE 4-4

Organ-Specific Listing of Commonly Used Medications

Central Nervous System (Neurology and Psychiatry)

Antianxiety and Sleep Agents (Anxiolytics and Hypnotics)

BENZODIAZEPINES

GENERIC NAME (BRAND NAME)	DOSAGE FORM	COMMON USES	COMMON/SEVERE ADVERSE EFFECTS	COMMENTS
alprazolam (Xanax)	PO	anxiety, panic disorder (attacks)	*Most common* – dizziness, sleepiness, delirium, NVDC, HA, slow heart rate, slow breathing, confusion *Rare but serious* – blood problems	Prolonged use can lead to dependence and a withdrawal syndrome when drugs are stopped.
clonazepam (Klonopin)	PO	panic disorder, epilepsy	↓	↓
diazepam (Valium)	PO, INJ	anxiety, epilepsy, alcohol withdrawal		
lorazepam (Ativan)	PO, INJ	anxiety, status epilepticus		
flurazepam (Dalmane)	PO	insomnia		
quazepam (Doral)	PO	insomnia		
temazepam (Restoril)	PO	insomnia	↓	↓

NONBENZODIAZEPINES

GENERIC NAME (BRAND NAME)	DOSAGE FORM	COMMON USES	COMMON/SEVERE ADVERSE EFFECTS	COMMENTS
buspirone (BuSpar)	PO	anxiety	*Most common* – dizziness, drowsiness, N, HA, nervousness	Dependence less likely than for benzodiazepines.
eszopiclone (Lunesta)	PO	insomnia	*Most common* – dry mouth, dizziness, hallucinations	↓
ramelteon (Rozerem)	PO	insomnia	*Most common* – drowsiness, dizziness, N, fatigue, HA	
zaleplon (Sonata)	PO	insomnia	*Most common* – memory loss	
zolpidem (Ambien)	PO	insomnia	*Most common* – dizziness, lethargy	↓

TABLE 4-4 (continued)

Organ-Specific Listing of Commonly Used Medications

Central Nervous System (Neurology and Psychiatry) [continued]

Antidepressant Agents (for depression, also used in mania and bipolar disorder)

GENERIC NAME (BRAND NAME)	DOSAGE FORM	COMMON USES	COMMON/SEVERE ADVERSE EFFECTS	COMMENTS
SELECTIVE SEROTONIN REUPTAKE INHIBITORS (SSRIs)				
citalopram (Celexa)	PO	depression	*Most common* – insomnia, N, tremor, nervousness, sweating, dry mouth, somnolence, weight loss	Discontinue therapy by gradually decreasing dose to avoid side effects.
escitalopram (Lexapro)	PO	depression, anxiety		
fluoxetine (Prozac)	PO	depression, OCD, panic disorder, bulimia		
paroxetine (Paxil)	PO	depression, OCD, anxiety, panic disorder		
sertraline (Zoloft)	PO	depression, OCD, panic disorder, anxiety		
TRICYCLIC ANTIDEPRESSANTS				
amitriptyline (Elavil)	PO, INJ	depression, pain of nerve origin (neuropathic pain)	*Most common* – AC, OH, sedation, confusion, weight gain, dizziness, heart problems	Dangerous in overdose.
imipramine (Tofranil)	PO	depression, childhood bedwetting	*Most common* – AC, OH, sedation, confusion, weight gain, dizziness, heart problems	Dangerous in overdose.
OTHER ANTIDEPRESSANTS				
bupropion (Wellbutrin)	PO	depression, smoking cessation	*Most common* – tremors, agitation, confusion, AC, dizziness *Rare but serious* – seizures	Zyban is trade name of smoking cessation product.
duloxetine (Cymbalta)	PO	depression, nerve pain, incontinence	*Most common* – insomnia, somnolence, dizziness, NC, dry mouth, anorexia	
mirtazapine (Remeron)	PO	depression	*Most common* – AC, somnolence, weight gain, OH *Rare but serious* – blood problems	
nefazodone (Serzone)	PO	depression	*Most common* – NC, dry mouth, somnolence, dizziness, confusion *Rare but serious* – liver damage	
trazodone (Desyrel)	PO	depression	*Most common* – drowsiness, dizziness, weight gain, blurred vision, OH *Rare but serious* – heart problems, painful erection	
venlafaxine (Effexor)	PO	depression, anxiety	*Most common* – N, sedation, dizziness, anxiety, insomnia, anorexia, dry mouth	Do not abruptly discontinue.

TABLE 4-4 (continued)

Organ-Specific Listing of Commonly Used Medications

Central Nervous System (Neurology and Psychiatry) [continued]

Antipsychotic Agents (for schizophrenia and other psychotic disorders)

GENERIC NAME (BRAND NAME)	DOSAGE FORM	COMMON USES	COMMON/SEVERE ADVERSE EFFECTS	COMMENTS
aripiprazole (Abilify)	PO	schizophrenia, bipolar mania	*Most common* – sedation, weight gain	
chlorpromazine (Thorazine)	PO, INJ, Supp	schizophrenia, bipolar disorder, vomiting	*Most common* – sedation, EPS, AC, OH	
clozapine (Clozaril)	PO	schizophrenia	*Most common* – sedation, dizziness, AC, heart problems , salivation *Rare but serious* – blood problems, seizures	Reserved for patients not responding to other therapy. Frequent blood tests required.
haloperidol (Haldol)	PO, INJ	schizophrenia, hyperactivity	*Most common* – EPS *Rare but serious* – heart problems	
olanzapine (Zyprexa)	PO, INJ	schizophrenia, bipolar disorder	*Most common* – sedation, agitation, AC, dizziness, weight gain	
quetiapine (Seroquel)	PO	schizophrenia, bipolar mania	*Most common* – sedation, OH, weight gain	
risperidone (Risperdal)	PO, INJ	schizophrenia, bipolar mania	*Most common* – agitation, AC, insomnia, nervousness, heart palpitations, weight gain	
ziprasidone (Geodon)	PO, INJ	schizophrenia, bipolar mania, acute agitation	*Most common* – sedation, EPS, OH *Rare but serious* – heart problems	

Antiparkinsonian Agents (for Parkinson's Disease)

GENERIC NAME (BRAND NAME)	DOSAGE FORM	COMMON USES	COMMON/SEVERE ADVERSE EFFECTS	COMMENTS
benztropine (Cogentin)	PO, INJ	Used to treat EPS induced by drugs for Parkinson's disease	*Most common* – AC, heart problems	
entacapone (Comtan)	PO	Used with levodopa/ carbidopa for Parkinson's disease	*Most common* – abnormal movements, OH, NVD, urine discoloration	Avoid abruptly discontinuing.
levodopa/ carbidopa (Sinemet)	PO	Parkinson's disease	*Most common* – NV, anorexia, OH, abnormal movements	
pergolide (Permax)	PO	Used with levodopa/ carbidopa for Parkinson's disease	*Most common* – abnormal movements, dizziness, sedation, OH, NC, hallucinations	
pramipexole (Mirapex)	PO	Parkinson's disease	*Most common* – OH, hallucinations, dizziness, sedation, N	

TABLE 4-4 (continued)

Organ-Specific Listing of Commonly Used Medications

Central Nervous System (Neurology and Psychiatry) [continued]

Antiparkinsonian Agents (for Parkinson's Disease) [continued]

GENERIC NAME (BRAND NAME)	DOSAGE FORM	COMMON USES	COMMON/SEVERE ADVERSE EFFECTS	COMMENTS
ropinirole (Requip)	PO	Parkinson's disease	*Most common* – OH, hallucinations, dizziness, sedation, N	
selegiline (Eldepryl)	PO	Used with levodopa/ carbidopa for Parkinson's disease	*Most common* – N, dizziness, dry mouth, confusion, hallucinations	Even though this agent is a monoamine oxidase inhibitor, patients can eat a normal diet if daily doses are less than 10 mg.

Drugs for Alzheimer's Disease

donepezil (Aricept)	PO	Alzheimer disease	*Most common* – NVD, anorexia, dizziness *Rare but serious* – slow heart rate, heart problems	Initiate therapy at low doses and slowly increase dose to lessen GI effects.
galantamine (Reminyl)	PO	Alzheimer disease	*Most common* – NVD, anorexia, dizziness *Rare but serious* – slow heart rate, heart problems	↓
rivastigmine (Exelon)	PO	Alzheimer disease	*Most common* – NVD, anorexia, dizziness *Rare but serious* – slow heart rate, heart problems	
memantine (Namenda)	PO	Alzheimer disease	*Most common* – dizziness, HA	

Centrally Acting Pain Medicines (mostly narcotic analgesics)

hydrocodone with APAP (example: Lortab, Vicodin)	PO	analgesic (pain relief)	*Most common* – sedation, dizziness, NC *Occur with higher doses* – slowed breathing, slowed heart rate	Physical dependence and withdrawal can occur with all opiates (in the same drug class as heroin).
morphine (example: MS Contin)	PO, INJ, supp	analgesic	↓	↓
propoxyphene with APAP (example: Darvocet-N)	PO	analgesic		
oxycodone with APAP (example: Percocet, Tylox)	PO	analgesic		
APAP with codeine (example: Tylenol #3)	PO	analgesic	*Most common* – NC, allergic and skin reactions, drowsiness	
tramadol (Ultram)	PO	analgesic	*Most common* – NC, dizziness, sedation, restlessness	Not an opiate

TABLE 4-4 (continued)

Organ-Specific Listing of Commonly Used Medications

Central Nervous System (Neurology and Psychiatry) [continued]

Drugs for Migraines

GENERIC NAME (BRAND NAME)	DOSAGE FORM	COMMON USES	COMMON/SEVERE ADVERSE EFFECTS	COMMENTS
eletriptan (Relpax)	PO	migraine	*Most common* – dizziness, flushing, tingling and pressure sensations throughout body *Rare but serious* – heart attack	
sumatriptan (Imitrex)	PO, INJ, nasal spray	migraine	*Most common* – dizziness, flushing, tingling and pressure sensations throughout body *Rare but serious* – heart attack	

Antiepileptic Medications (to prevent seizures)

GENERIC NAME (BRAND NAME)	DOSAGE FORM	COMMON USES	COMMON/SEVERE ADVERSE EFFECTS	COMMENTS
carbamazepine (Tegretol)	PO	epilepsy (seizures)	*Most common* – N, drowsiness, dizziness *Rare but serious* – blood problems, liver problems, severe rash	Do not use in patients with histories of bone marrow suppression and related blood disorders.
gabapentin (Neurontin)	PO	adjuvant (add-on) therapy for seizures, nerve pain	*Most common* – sleepiness, dizziness, dry mouth, blurred vision	
phenytoin (Dilantin)	PO, INJ	epilepsy	*Most common but dose-related* – nystagmus (eye deviations), abnormal movements, dizziness *Rare but serious* – severe rash, and blood, liver, heart problems	Blood levels must be monitored to avoid toxicities. Do not interchange tablets and capsules or change brands without prescriber's knowledge.
pregabalin (Lyrica)	PO	seizures, nerve pain	*Most common* – dizziness, somnolence, edema, dry mouth, blurred vision, weight gain	
valproic acid (Depakote)	PO, INJ	epilepsy, mania	*Most common* – somnolence, dizziness, ND, hair loss *Rare but serious* – liver, pancreas, and blood problems	Avoid in pregnancy.

Drugs for Attention-Deficit/Hyperactivity Disorder (ADHD)

GENERIC NAME (BRAND NAME)	DOSAGE FORM	COMMON USES	COMMON/SEVERE ADVERSE EFFECTS	COMMENTS
amphetamine mixture (Adderall)	PO	ADHD, narcolepsy	*Most common* – decreased appetite, fast heart rate, restlessness, high blood pressure	High abuse potential. May slow growth in children.
atomoxetine (Strattera)	PO	ADHD	*Most common* – decreased appetite, dizziness	May slow growth in children.
methylphenidate (Ritalin, Concerta)	PO	ADHD, narcolepsy	*Most common* – decreased appetite, restlessness	Can induce dependency and a withdrawal syndrome. May slow growth in children.

Antiemetics (to stop vomiting)

GENERIC NAME (BRAND NAME)	DOSAGE FORM	COMMON USES	COMMON/SEVERE ADVERSE EFFECTS	COMMENTS
metoclopramide (Reglan)	PO, INJ	NV due to chemotherapy, diabetic gastroparesis	*Most common* – EPS, drowsiness, dizziness *Rare but serious* – neuroleptic malignant syndrome, depression	
granisetron (Kytril)	PO, INJ	NV due to chemotherapy, radiation, surgery	*Most common* – HA, C	

TABLE 4-4 (continued)

Organ-Specific Listing of Commonly Used Medications

Central Nervous System (Neurology and Psychiatry) [continued]

Antiemetics (to stop vomiting) [continued]

GENERIC NAME (BRAND NAME)	DOSAGE FORM	COMMON USES	COMMON/SEVERE ADVERSE EFFECTS	COMMENTS
ondansetron (Zofran)	PO, INJ	NV due to chemotherapy, radiation, surgery	*Most common* – sedation, HA	
prochlorperazine (Compazine)	PO, INJ, supp	NV	*Most common* – EPS, sedation	
trimethobenzamide (Tigan)	PO, INJ, supp	NV	*Most common* – sedation, dizziness, abnormal movements	

Eye, Ear, Nose, and Throat Agents (Ophthalmology and Otolaryngology)

GENERIC NAME (BRAND NAME)	DOSAGE FORM	COMMON USES	COMMON/SEVERE ADVERSE EFFECTS	COMMENTS
Antihistamines				
cetirizine (Zyrtec)	PO	allergic rhinitis, chronic urticaria (hives)	*Most common* – sedation	
desloratadine (Clarinex)	PO	allergic rhinitis, chronic urticaria		
fexofenadine (Allegra)	PO	allergic rhinitis, chronic urticaria		
loratadine (Claritin)	PO	allergic rhinitis		Available OTC.
Nasal Corticosteroids				
fluticasone (Flonase)	nasal spray	rhinitis	*Most common* – sore throat, nosebleed, cough	
mometasone (Nasonex)	nasal spray	allergic rhinitis		Can worsen existing breathing problems.
triamcinolone (Nasacort)	nasal spray	allergic rhinitis		
Ophthalmics (for the eye)				
dorzolamide (Trusopt)	eye drop	elevated intraocular pressure (glaucoma)	*Most common* – eye irritation, bitter taste	
latanoprost (Xalatan)	eye drop	elevated intraocular pressure (glaucoma)	*Most common* – eye irritation, brown pigmentation of the iris	
timolol (Timoptic)	eye drop	elevated intraocular pressure	*Most common* – eye redness, slow heart rate, low blood pressure	

TABLE 4-4 (continued)

Organ-Specific Listing of Commonly Used Medications

Respiratory Agents (for the lungs and airways)

Inhaled Corticosteroids

GENERIC NAME (BRAND NAME)	DOSAGE FORM	COMMON USES	COMMON/SEVERE ADVERSE EFFECTS	COMMENTS
fluticasone (Flovent)	oral inhalation	asthma	*Most common* – sore throat, nasal congestion, oral candidiasis (thrush, fungal infection of mouth)	
triamcinolone (Azmacort)	oral inhalation	asthma	*Most common* – sore throat, nasal congestion, oral candidiasis (thrush, fungal infection of mouth)	

Beta Agonists

albuterol	PO, oral inhalation	asthma	*Most common* – Fast heart rate, tremor, throat irritation	
salmeterol (Serevent)	oral inhalation	asthma, COPD	*Most common* – Fast heart rate, tremor, throat irritation	

Other

dextromethorphan	PO	cough – for suppression	*Most common* – drowsiness, dizziness	Available OTC.
guaifenesin	PO	cough – to loosen mucus	*Common* – NV	Some products available OTC.
ipratropium (Atrovent)	oral inhalation, nasal spray	COPD (bronchitis, emphysema)	*Most common* – cough, mouth/nose dryness, nervousness, nose bleed	
montelukast (Singulair)	PO	asthma, allergic rhinitis	*Most common* – indigestion	
tiotropium (Spiriva)	oral inhalation	COPD	*Most common* – dry mouth	

Gastroenterologic Agents (for the gastrointestinal tract, liver, and gallbladder)

Histamine-2 H₂ Antagonists

famotidine (Pepcid)	PO, INJ	PUD, GERD	*Most common* – HA, dizziness	Some strengths available OTC.
nizatidine (Axid)	PO	PUD, GERD	↓	↓
ranitidine (Zantac)	PO, INJ	PUD, GERD		

Proton Pump Inhibitors

esomeprazole (Nexium)	PO	erosive esophagitis, GERD, *Helicobacter pylori* infection	*Most common* – HA, dizziness	
lansoprazole (Prevacid)	PO, INJ	PUD, GERD, esophagitis, *H. pylori* infection	↓	
omeprazole (Prilosec)	PO	PUD, GERD, esophagitis		
pantoprazole (Protonix)	PO, INJ	esophagitis, GERD		
rabeprazole (AcipHex)	PO	PUD, GERD, *H. pylori* infection		

TABLE 4-4 (continued)

Organ-Specific Listing of Commonly Used Medications

Gastroenterologic Agents (for the gastrointestinal tract, liver, and gallbladder) [continued]

Other

GENERIC NAME (BRAND NAME)	DOSAGE FORM	COMMON USES	COMMON/SEVERE ADVERSE EFFECTS	COMMENTS
infliximab (Remicade)	INJ	Crohn disease, rheumatoid arthritis	*Most common* – rash, HA, SOB (infusion-related reactions) *Rare but serious* – rare infections, heart failure	Should be administered in a health-care setting.
sucralfate (Carafate)	PO	PUD	*Most common* – C	
tegaserod (Zelnorm)	PO	irritable bowel syndrome	*Most common* – D	

Endocrinologic Agents (for the pituitary, thyroid, and adrenal glands, and the pancreas)

Drugs for Diabetes

GENERIC NAME (BRAND NAME)	DOSAGE FORM	COMMON USES	COMMON/SEVERE ADVERSE EFFECTS	COMMENTS
glimepiride (Amaryl)	PO	type 2 diabetes	*Most common* – low blood glucose, N, heartburn	
glipizide (Glucotrol)	PO	type 2 diabetes		
glyburide (Diaßeta)	PO	type 2 diabetes		
insulin	INJ, nasal spray	type 1 and type 2 diabetes	*Most common* – low blood glucose, injection-site reactions	Available in many different forms, some long-acting, some short-acting.
metformin (Glucophage)	PO	type 2 diabetes	*Most common* – D, N, V, flatulence (gas) *Rare but serious* – lactic acidosis	Avoid in patients with kidney disease or CHF.
pioglitazone (Actos)	PO	type 2 diabetes	*Most common* – edema (fluid retention)	Monitor liver function. Avoid in patients with moderate to severe CHF.
rosiglitazone (Avandia)	PO	type 2 diabetes		
pramlintide (Symlin)	SQ	type 1 or 2 diabetes	*Most common* – Nausea, anorexia, vomiting, fatigue, inflicted injury, headache *Rare but serious* – severe hypoglycemia	Contraindicated in patients with a confirmed diagnosis of gastroparesis; should not be considered for patients who are taking drugs that alter GI motility or slow the intestinal absorption of nutrients.
exenatide (Byetta)	SQ	type 2 diabetes	*Most common* – nausea, vomiting, diarrhea, feeling jittery, dizziness, headache, and dyspepsia *Rare but serious* – Not recommended in patients with severe gastrointestinal disease, including gastroparesis, a complication of diabetes	Administered in the thigh, abdomen, or upper arm at any time within 60 minutes before morning and evening meals; should not be administered after a meal.

TABLE 4-4 (continued)

Organ-Specific Listing of Commonly Used Medications

Endocrinologic Agents (for the pituitary, thyroid, and adrenal glands, and the pancreas) [continued]
Corticosteroids

GENERIC NAME (BRAND NAME)	DOSAGE FORM	COMMON USES	COMMON/SEVERE ADVERSE EFFECTS	COMMENTS
dexamethasone	PO, INJ	anti-inflammatory agents; used in wide variety of conditions	*Most common* – insomnia, nervousness, increased appetite, indigestion *Rare but serious* – diabetes, cataracts, glaucoma, immunosuppression, PUD	Do not abruptly discontinue if taking high doses for prolonged period of time.
hydrocortisone	PO, INJ	anti-inflammatory agents; used in wide variety of conditions	↓	↓
methylprednisolone	PO, INJ	anti-inflammatory agents; used in wide variety of conditions		
prednisone	PO	anti-inflammatory agents; used in wide variety of conditions		
triamcinolone	PO, INJ	anti-inflammatory agents; used in wide variety of conditions		

Estrogens and Progestins (Sex Hormones)

GENERIC NAME (BRAND NAME)	DOSAGE FORM	COMMON USES	COMMON/SEVERE ADVERSE EFFECTS	COMMENTS
conjugated estrogens (Premarin)	PO, INJ	menopausal symptoms	*Most common* – HA, dizziness, N, changes in vaginal bleeding and patterns, fluid retention *Rare but serious* – blood clots (including heart attack and pulmonary embolism)	May increase risk for endometrial cancer in postmenopausal women.
estradiol (example: Estrace, Vivelle, Climara)	PO, INJ, TOP	menopausal symptoms, atrophic vaginitis	↓	May increase risk for endometrial cancer in postmenopausal women.
oral contraceptives (usually combine estrogen and progestin)	PO, TOP, vaginal	birth control, emergency contraception (prevention of pregnancy after intercourse), menstrual problems		Smoking increases risk of cardiovascular side effects.
medroxy-progesterone (Provera)	PO	menstrual and uterine problems	*Most common* – edema (swelling), breakthrough menstrual bleeding, changes in menstrual cycle (including no periods) *Rare but serious* – blood clots	
raloxifene (Evista)	PO	osteoporosis	*Most common* – hot flushes, leg cramps *Rare but serious* – blood clots	

Other

GENERIC NAME (BRAND NAME)	DOSAGE FORM	COMMON USES	COMMON/SEVERE ADVERSE EFFECTS	COMMENTS
levothyroxine (Synthroid)	PO, INJ	thyroid-replacement therapy	*Dose-related (dose too high)* – nervousness, fast heart rate, HA, insomnia, fever, weight loss, increased appetite, D	Do not change brands without prescriber's knowledge.

TABLE 4-4 (continued)

Organ-Specific Listing of Commonly Used Medications

Cardiac Agents (for the heart)
Angiotensin-Converting Enzyme (ACE) Inhibitors

GENERIC NAME (BRAND NAME)	DOSAGE FORM	COMMON USES	COMMON/SEVERE ADVERSE EFFECTS	COMMENTS
benazepril (Lotensin)	PO	HTN	*Most common* – dizziness, cough *Rare but serious* – angioedema (severe allergic reaction causing throat swelling)	Avoid during second and third trimester of pregnancy. Monitor for hyperkalemia (high blood potassium levels).
enalapril (Vasotec)	PO, INJ	HTN, CHF		
fosinopril (Monopril)	PO	HTN, CHF		
lisinopril (Zestril, Prinivil)	PO	HTN, CHF, acute MI (heart attack)		
quinapril (Accupril)	PO	HTN, CHF		
ramipril (Altace)	PO	HTN, CHF, prevention of cardiovascular disease in high risk patients		

Angiotensin Receptor Blockers (ARBs)

irbesartan (Avapro)	PO	HTN, kidney disease in diabetic patients	*Most common* – cough (less common than with ACE inhibitors)	Avoid during second and third trimester of pregnancy. Monitor for hyperkalemia (high blood potassium levels).
losartan (Cozaar)	PO	HTN, kidney disease in diabetic patients		
valsartan (Diovan)	PO	HTN, CHF		

Calcium Channel Blockers

amlodipine (Norvasc)	PO	HTN, angina	*Most common* – peripheral edema (swelling of feet, ankles), low blood pressure, dizziness, C *Rare but serious* – heart problems (especially with verapamil)	

TABLE 4-4 (continued)

Organ-Specific Listing of Commonly Used Medications

Cardiac Agents (for the heart) [continued]
Calcium Channel Blockers (continued)

GENERIC NAME (BRAND NAME)	DOSAGE FORM	COMMON USES	COMMON/SEVERE ADVERSE EFFECTS	COMMENTS
diltiazem (Cardizem, Tiazac)	PO, INJ	HTN, AF, angina, PSVT	*Most common* – peripheral edema (swelling of feet, ankles), low blood pressure, dizziness, C *Rare but serious* – heart problems (especially with verapamil)	
felodipine (Plendil)	PO	HTN		
nifedipine (Procardia, Adalat)	PO	HTN, angina		
verapamil (Calan, Verelan)	PO, INJ	angina, HTN, PSVT, AF		

Other

amiodarone (Cordarone, Pacerone)	PO, INJ	arrhythmias (abnormal heart rhythms)	*Most common* – malaise, tremor, NVC, visual problems, slow heart rate, sensitivity to sun *Rare but serious* – lung problems, arrhythmias, liver problems, eye problems, thyroid problems	
digoxin (Lanoxin)	PO, INJ	CHF, AF	*Dose-related (dose too high)* – anorexia, N, V, drowsiness, slow heart rate, confusion, visual changes	Drug concentrations in the blood should be monitored to avoid toxicity.

Vascular Agents (for the blood vessels)
Beta-Blockers

atenolol (Tenormin)	PO, INJ	HTN, angina, acute MI	*Most common* – slow heart rate, dizziness, fatigue, wheezing	
metoprolol (Lopressor, Toprol)	PO, INJ	HTN, angina, MI, CHF		
propranolol (Inderal)	PO, INJ	HTN, angina, migraine HA		

Other Antiadrenergic Agents

carvedilol (Coreg)	PO	HTN, CHF	*Most common* – OH, D, dizziness, slow heart rate *Rare but serious* – liver problems	
clonidine (Catapres)	PO, TOP, INJ	HTN, opiate withdrawal, smoking cessation	*Most common* – drowsiness, dizziness, dry mouth, constipation	Do not abruptly discontinue therapy.

TABLE 4-4 (continued)

Organ-Specific Listing of Commonly Used Medications

Vascular Agents (for the blood vessels) [continued]
Other Antiadrenergic Agents (continued)

GENERIC NAME (BRAND NAME)	DOSAGE FORM	COMMON USES	COMMON/SEVERE ADVERSE EFFECTS	COMMENTS
doxazosin (Cardura)	PO	HTN, benign prostatic hypertrophy	*Most common* – OH, dizziness, HA, fatigue	Do not abruptly discontinue therapy.
labetalol (Trandate, Normodyne)	PO, INJ	HTN	*Most common* – dizziness, N, OH *Rare but serious* – liver problems	
terazosin (Hytrin)	PO	HTN, benign prostatic hypertrophy	*Most common* – OH, dizziness, HA, fatigue, edema	

Vasodilators

isosorbide mononitrate (Imdur, Monoket)	PO	angina	*Most common* – HA, dizziness, OH	
nesiritide (Natrecor)	INJ	severe CHF	*Most common* – low blood pressure, dizziness, N	
nitroglycerin (example: Nitrostat, Nitro-Dur, Transderm Nitro)	PO, INJ, TOP	angina	*Most common* – OH, HA, flushing, dizziness, weakness	Sublingual tablets are placed under the tongue.

Antihyperlipidemic Agents (to lower cholesterol)

atorvastatin (Lipitor)	PO	hyperlipidemias	*Most common* – flatulence (gas) *Rare but serious* – muscle problems, liver problems	Contraindicated during pregnancy.
fluvastatin (Lescol)	PO	hyperlipidemias	↓	↓
lovastatin (Mevacor)	PO	hyperlipidemias	↓	↓
pravastatin (Pravachol)	PO	hyperlipidemias	↓	↓
rosuvastatin (Crestor)	PO	hyperlipidemias	↓	↓
simvastatin (Zocor)	PO	hyperlipidemias	↓	↓
ezetimibe (Zetia)	PO	hyperlipidemias	*Rare* – D	

TABLE 4-4 (continued)

Organ-Specific Listing of Commonly Used Medications

Vascular Agents (for the blood vessels) [continued]
Antihyperlipidemic Agents (to lower cholesterol) [continued]

GENERIC NAME (BRAND NAME)	DOSAGE FORM	COMMON USES	COMMON/SEVERE ADVERSE EFFECTS	COMMENTS
fenofibrate (TriCor)	PO	hyperlipidemias	*Most common* – NC *Rare but serious* – liver problems, gallbladder problems (gallstones)	
gemfibrozil (Lopid)	PO	high triglyceride levels	*Most common* – dyspepsia (upset stomach), abdominal pain, DNV *Rare but serious* – gallbladder problems	

Anticoagulant and Antiplatelet Agents (prevent blood clots)

* APPLICABLE TO ALL ANTICOAGULANT AND ANTIPLATELET AGENTS: Bleeding is the major risk with all anticoagulant and antiplatelet agents. It can occur from any body site and range from mild to severe. It is usually dose-related. The effects of the drug in blood should be monitored for abciximab, eptifibatide, heparin, tirofiban, and warfarin.

GENERIC NAME (BRAND NAME)	DOSAGE FORM	COMMON USES	COMMON/SEVERE ADVERSE EFFECTS	COMMENTS
abciximab (ReoPro)	INJ	acute MI		* see comment above
aspirin	PO	prevention of stroke, MI		* see comment above
clopidogrel (Plavix)	PO	recent MI or stroke		* see comment above
dalteparin (Fragmin)	INJ	acute MI, prevention of DVT		* see comment above
enoxaparin (Lovenox)	INJ	DVT, PE, acute MI		* see comment above
eptifibatide (Integrilin)	INJ	acute MI		* see comment above
heparin	INJ	DVT, PE		* see comment above
pentoxifylline (Trental)	PO	intermittent claudication (poor blood flow to limbs)		* see comment above
tenecteplase (TNKase)	INJ	acute MI ("clot buster")		* see comment above
tinzaparin (Innohep)	INJ	DVT		* see comment above
tirofiban (Aggrastat)	INJ	acute MI		* see comment above
warfarin (Coumadin)	PO, INJ	prevention and treatment of DVT, PE; atrial fibrillation		Avoid warfarin during pregnancy.

Renal Agents (for the kidneys)

GENERIC NAME (BRAND NAME)	DOSAGE FORM	COMMON USES	COMMON/SEVERE ADVERSE EFFECTS	COMMENTS
furosemide (Lasix)	PO, INJ	HTN, edema, CHF	*Most common* – electrolyte (sodium, potassium, chloride) imbalance, OH, sun sensitivity *Rare but serious* – hearing loss	
hydrochlorothiazide	PO	HTN, edema	*Most common* – OH, low blood potassium, sun sensitivity	Often abbreviated HCTZ.
spironolactone (Aldactone)	PO	CHF, HTN	*Most common* – high blood potassium, gynecomastia (breast enlargement in men)	

TABLE 4-4 (continued)

Organ-Specific Listing of Commonly Used Medications

Renal Agents (for the kidneys) [continued]

GENERIC NAME (BRAND NAME)	DOSAGE FORM	COMMON USES	COMMON/SEVERE ADVERSE EFFECTS	COMMENTS
torsemide (Demadex)	PO, INJ	CHF, HTN, edema	*Most common* – electrolyte (sodium, potassium, chloride) imbalance, OH, sun sensitivity *Rare but serious* – hearing loss	
triamterene/HCTZ (Maxzide, Dyazide)	PO	edema, HTN, CHF	*Most common* – electrolyte imbalances, sun sensitivity	

Genitourinary Agents

GENERIC NAME (BRAND NAME)	DOSAGE FORM	COMMON USES	COMMON/SEVERE ADVERSE EFFECTS	COMMENTS
dutasteride (Avodart)	PO	benign prostatic hyperplasia	*Most common* – decreased libido	Do not use in women or children. Pregnant women should not even handle the drug.
finasteride (Propecia, Proscar)	PO	benign prostatic hyperplasia, male pattern baldness	*Most common* – decreased libido	Do not use in women or children. Pregnant women should not even handle the drug.
darifenacin (Enablex)	PO	urinary incontinence	*Most common* – AC, C	
oxybutynin (Ditropan)	PO, TOP			
solifenacin (Vesicare)	PO			
tolterodine (Detrol)	PO			
trospium (Sanctura)	PO			
sildenafil (Viagra)	PO	erectile dysfunction	*Most common* – HA, flushing, dyspepsia (upset stomach), visual changes *Rare but serious* – heart problems (including death) in men who already have cardiac disease	
tadalafil (Cialis)	PO			
vardenafil (Levitra)	PO			

TABLE 4-4 (continued)

Organ-Specific Listing of Commonly Used Medications

Bone and Joint Agents (including pain drugs that act peripherally)
Nonsteroidal Anti-Inflammatory Drugs (NSAIDs)

GENERIC NAME (BRAND NAME)	DOSAGE FORM	COMMON USES	COMMON/SEVERE ADVERSE EFFECTS	COMMENTS
diclofenac (Voltaren)	PO	pain, fever, inflammation (i.e. arthritis)	*Most common* – abdominal pain, prolonged bleeding time *Rare but serious* – GI ulceration, kidney problems	
ibuprofen (Motrin)	PO, INJ	pain, fever, inflammation (i.e. arthritis)	↓	
ketorolac (Toradol)	PO	moderately severe acute pain	↓	
nabumetone (Relafen)	PO	pain, fever, inflammation (i.e. arthritis)	↓	
naproxen (Naprosyn)	PO	↓	↓	
oxaprozin (Daypro)	PO	↓	↓	

COX-2 Inhibitors

celecoxib (Celebrex)	PO	pain, inflammation (i.e. arthritis)	*Most common* – abdominal pain, prolonged bleeding time *Rare but serious* – cardiovascular events; kidney problems	The COX-2 inhibitors are regarded as less damaging to the GI tract than the NSAIDs, but they have been associated with serious cardiovascular adverse events, including myocardial infarction (heart attack) and sudden (unexplained) cardiac death.

Other Analgesics

acetaminophen (Tylenol)	PO, Supp	pain, fever	*Rare but serious* – liver problems (especially in overdose)	Often abbreviated APAP.
carisoprodol (Soma)	PO	muscle pain	*Most common* – drowsiness, dizziness	
cyclobenzaprine (Flexeril)	PO	muscle pain	*Most common* – AC, drowsiness, dizziness	

TABLE 4-4 (continued)

Organ-Specific Listing of Commonly Used Medications

Bone and Joint Agents (including pain drugs that act peripherally) [continued]

GENERIC NAME (BRAND NAME)	DOSAGE FORM	COMMON USES	COMMON/SEVERE ADVERSE EFFECTS	COMMENTS
Drugs for Osteoporosis				
alendronate (Fosamax)	PO	osteoporosis	*Most common* – esophageal irritation (prevent by taking with full glass of water and not lying down after taking	
ibandronate (Boniva)	PO	osteoporosis		
risedronate (Actonel)	PO	osteoporosis		
calcitonin (Miacalcin)	INJ, nasal spray	osteoporosis	*Most common* – injection site reactions, nasal irritation (nasal spray), flushing of face/hands, N	
Drugs for Gout				
allopurinol (Zyloprim)	PO	gout	*Most common* – rash (stop drug – can become severe) *Rare but serious* – liver problems, severe rash, kidney problems	
colchicine	PO, INJ	gout	*Most common* – NVD *Rare but serious* – blood problems	

TABLE 4-4 (continued)

Organ-Specific Listing of Commonly Used Medications

Anti-Infective Agents (for bacterial, viral, and fungal infections)

* APPLICABLE TO ALL ANTIBIOTICS: Antibiotic choice is determined by the infecting microorganism – if unknown, then the most likely infecting organism(s) is targeted. Organisms can develop resistance to antibiotics, requiring the use of different antibiotics. Antibiotics are ineffective against viral infections.

Penicillins

GENERIC NAME (BRAND NAME)	DOSAGE FORM	COMMON USES	COMMON/SEVERE ADVERSE EFFECTS	COMMENTS
amoxicillin (Amoxil)	PO	infections of ear, nose, throat, skin, lungs, urinary tract	*Most common* – allergic reactions, D	* see comment above
amoxicillin/ clavulanic acid (Augmentin)	PO	infections of ear, nose, throat, skin, lungs, urinary tract		* see comment above
piperacillin/ tazobactam (Zosyn)	INJ	intra-abdominal infections, pneumonia		* see comment above
ticarcillin/ clavulanic acid (Timentin)	INJ	intra-abdominal infections, pneumonia		* see comment above

Cephalosporins

cefaclor (Ceclor)	PO	otitis media (ear infection), UTI, bronchitis	*Most common* – allergic reactions, D (including a severe form called pseudomembranous colitis)	* see comment above
cephalexin (Keflex)	PO	otitis media, UTI		* see comment above
cefazolin (Ancef)	INJ	surgical prophylaxis, pneumonia, UTI		* see comment above
cefprozil (Cefzil)	PO	otitis media, sinusitis		* see comment above
loracarbef (Lorabid)	PO	otitis media, pneumonia, UTI		* see comment above
cefuroxime (Ceftin, Zinacef)	PO, INJ	otitis media, UTI		* see comment above
cefotetan (Cefotan)	INJ	intra-abdominal infections		* see comment above
cefpodoxime (Vantin)	PO	pneumonia, gonorrhea		* see comment above
cefixime (Suprax)	PO	UTI, otitis media		* see comment above
cefoperazone (Cefobid)	INJ	pneumonia, intra-abdominal infections		* see comment above
cefotaxime (Claforan)	INJ	pneumonia, intra-abdominal infections		* see comment above

TABLE 4-4 (continued)

Organ-Specific Listing of Commonly Used Medications

Anti-Infective Agents (for bacterial, viral, and fungal infections) [continued]

* APPLICABLE TO ALL ANTIBIOTICS: Antibiotic choice is determined by the infecting microorganism – if unknown, then the most likely infecting organism(s) is targeted. Organisms can develop resistance to antibiotics, requiring the use of different antibiotics. Antibiotics are ineffective against viral infections.

Cephalosporins (continued)

GENERIC NAME (BRAND NAME)	DOSAGE FORM	COMMON USES	COMMON/SEVERE ADVERSE EFFECTS	COMMENTS
ceftazidime (Fortaz)	INJ	pneumonia	*Most common* – allergic reactions, D (including a severe form called pseudomembranous colitis)	* see comment above
ceftriaxone (Rocephin)	INJ	pneumonia, gonorrhea, meningitis		* see comment above
cefepime (Maxipime)	INJ	pneumonia		* see comment above

Macrolides and Ketolides

azithromycin (Zithromax)	PO, INJ	pneumonia, sinusitis	*Most common* – ND, abdominal pain (worse with erythromycin) *Rare but serious* – liver problems, heart problems, pseudomembranous colitis	* see comment above
clarithromycin (Biaxin)	PO	pneumonia, sinusitis, *H. pylori* infections		* see comment above
erythromycin	PO, INJ	upper respiratory tract infection, pneumonia		* see comment above
telithromycin (Ketek)	PO	pneumonia	*Most common* – ND, visual problems *Rare but serious* – pseudomembranous colitis, heart problems, liver problems	* see comment above

Quinolones

ciprofloxacin (Cipro)	PO, INJ	pneumonia, UTI	*Most common* – sun sensitivity *Rare but serious* – tendon rupture, heart problems, pseudomembranous colitis	* see comment above
gatifloxacin (Tequin)	PO, INJ	pneumonia, UTI	*Most common* – ND, abdominal pain (worse with erythromycin) *Rare but serious* – liver problems, heart problems, pseudomembranous colitis	* see comment above
gemifloxacin (Factive)	PO, INJ	pneumonia		* see comment above
levofloxacin (Levaquin)	PO, INJ	pneumonia, UTI		* see comment above
moxifloxacin (Avelox)	PO, INJ	pneumonia, sinusitis		* see comment above

TABLE 4-4 (continued)

Organ-Specific Listing of Commonly Used Medications

Anti-Infective Agents (for bacterial, viral, and fungal infections) [continued]

* APPLICABLE TO ALL ANTIBIOTICS: Antibiotic choice is determined by the infecting microorganism – if unknown, then the most likely infecting organism(s) is targeted. Organisms can develop resistance to antibiotics, requiring the use of different antibiotics. Antibiotics are ineffective against viral infections.

Other Antibiotics

GENERIC NAME (BRAND NAME)	DOSAGE FORM	COMMON USES	COMMON/SEVERE ADVERSE EFFECTS	COMMENTS
aztreonam (Azactam)	INJ	UTI, sepsis (blood infection)	*Most common* – rash, ND	* see comment above
clindamycin (Cleocin)	PO, INJ	intra-abdominal infections	*Most common* – D (can be severe)	* see comment above
gentamicin	INJ	sepsis, UTI	*Rare but serious* – kidney problems, ear problems	* see comment above Blood levels should be monitored.
imipenem/ cilastatin (Primaxin)	INJ	intra-abdominal infections, foot infections in diabetics	*Rare but serious* – seizures, pseudomembranous colitis	* see comment above
metronidazole (Flagyl)	PO, INJ	intra-abdominal infections, foot infections in diabetics	*Most common* – ND, metallic taste *Rare but serious* – seizures	* see comment above Avoid alcohol while taking.
tigecycline (Tygacil)	INJ	intra-abdominal infections, skin infections	*Most common* – NV *Rare but serious* – permanent tooth discoloration in infants, children	* see comment above Avoid in children < 8 years old and during pregnancy.
tobramycin (Nebcin)	INJ	sepsis, pneumonia	*Rare but serious* – kidney problems, ear problems	* see comment above Blood levels should be monitored.
trimethoprim/ sulfamethoxazole (Bactrim, Septra)	PO, INJ	UTI	*Most common* – NV, anorexia, allergic reactions	* see comment above
vancomycin (Vancocin)	PO, INJ	infections due to MRSA (methicillin-resistant *S. aureus*)	*Most common* – infusion-related reactions *Rare but serious* – kidney problems, ear problems, blood problems	* see comment above Blood levels should be monitored. Oral form of drug only for treatment of pseudomembranous colitis.

Antifungal Agents

GENERIC NAME (BRAND NAME)	DOSAGE FORM	COMMON USES	COMMON/SEVERE ADVERSE EFFECTS	COMMENTS
amphotericin B	INJ	severe systemic fungal infections	*Most common* – infusion reactions (fever, chills, NV, HA) *Rare but serious* – kidney problems (less risk with lipid formulations)	* see comment above Pretreatment with antihistamines, APAP, and corticosteroids helps lessen infusion reactions.
fluconazole (Diflucan)	PO, INJ	candidiasis, severe fungal infections	*Most common* – HA, N *Rare but serious* – liver damage, severe rash	* see comment above
itraconazole (Sporanox)	PO, INJ	severe fungal infections, toenail infections	*Most common* – N *Rare but serious* – CHF, liver damage	* see comment above Avoid in patients with CHF.
ketoconazole (Nizoral)	PO	severe fungal infections	*Most common* – NV *Rare but serious* – liver damage	* see comment above
terbinafine (Lamisil)	PO	severe fungal toenail infections	*Most common* – rash, D *Rare but serious* – liver damage	* see comment above

TABLE 4-4 (continued)

Organ-Specific Listing of Commonly Used Medications

Antiviral Agents

Antiretroviral Agents (for HIV infection)

PROTEASE INHIBITORS

All protease inhibitors can cause high blood sugar, including diabetes, and redistribution of body fat (buffalo hump), sometimes with cholesterol abnormalities. There are many drug interactions. Many PIs should be stored in the refrigerator.

GENERIC NAME (BRAND NAME)	DOSAGE FORM	COMMON USES	COMMON/SEVERE ADVERSE EFFECTS	COMMENTS
atazanavir (Reyataz)	PO	HIV (in combination with the nucleoside and non-nucleoside reverse transcriptase inhibitors)	*Most common* – N, sun sensitivity *Rare but serious* – heart rhythm problems, liver problems	
indinavir (Crixivan)	PO		*Most common* – N *Rare but serious* – kidney stones, liver problems, blood problems	
nelfinavir (Viracept)	PO		*Most common* – D	
ritonavir (Norvir)	PO		*Most common* – NVD, anorexia, abdominal pain *Rare but serious* – pancreas, liver problems	
saquinavir (Fortovase)	PO		*Most common* – indigestion	

NUCLEOSIDE REVERSE TRANSCRIPTASE INHIBITORS

GENERIC NAME (BRAND NAME)	DOSAGE FORM	COMMON USES	COMMON/SEVERE ADVERSE EFFECTS	COMMENTS
didanosine (Videx)	PO	HIV (in combination with a protease inhibitor). Lamivudine is also used for hepatitis B infection.	*Most common* – D, abdominal pain *Rare but serious* – pancreatitis, liver problems, lactic acidosis (build-up of lactic acid), peripheral neuropathy (pain, weakness, numbness in hands, feet)	Abbreviated ddI.
lamivudine (Epivir)	PO		*Rare but serious* – liver problems, lactic acidosis	Abbreviated 3TC.

TABLE 4-4 (continued)

Organ-Specific Listing of Commonly Used Medications

Antiviral Agents (continued)

Antiretroviral Agents (for HIV infection) [continued]

NUCLEOSIDE REVERSE TRANSCRIPTASE INHIBITORS (CONTINUED)

GENERIC NAME (BRAND NAME)	DOSAGE FORM	COMMON USES	COMMON/SEVERE ADVERSE EFFECTS	COMMENTS
stavudine (Zerit)	PO	HIV (in combination with a protease inhibitor). Lamivudine is also used for hepatitis B infection.	*Most common* – peripheral neuropathy (dose-related) *Rare but serious* – liver problems, lactic acidosis	Abbreviated d4T.
zalcitabine (Hivid)	PO		*Most common* – peripheral neuropathy *Rare but serious* – liver problems, lactic acidosis, pancreatitis	Abbreviated ddC.
zidovudine (Retrovir)	PO, INJ		*Most common* – NV, fatigue *Rare but serious* – blood problems, liver problems, lactic acidosis	Abbreviated AZT.

Other Antiviral Agents

GENERIC NAME (BRAND NAME)	DOSAGE FORM	COMMON USES	COMMON/SEVERE ADVERSE EFFECTS	COMMENTS
acyclovir (Zovirax)	PO, INJ	herpes, chickenpox	*Most common* – ND *Rare but serious* – kidney problems	
amantadine (Symmetrel)	PO	influenza A, Parkinson's disease	*Most common* – dizziness, insomnia, N, edema *Rare but serious* – suicide	Dangerous in overdose.
oseltamivir (Tamiflu)	PO	influenza A and B	*Most common* – NV	
ribavirin (Rebetol, Copegus)	PO, aerosol	hepatitis C (with interferon alfa), RSV in infants	*Most common* – anxiety, depression, fatigue *Rare but serious* – blood, heart problems, suicide	Contraindicated in pregnancy.
zanamivir (Relenza)	inhalation	influenza A and B	*Most common* – breathing problems	

TABLE 4-4 (continued)

Organ-Specific Listing of Commonly Used Medications

Oncolytic Agents (for cancers, both solid tumors and blood cancers)

Alkylating Agents and Platinum Compounds

GENERIC NAME (BRAND NAME)	DOSAGE FORM	COMMON USES	COMMON/SEVERE ADVERSE EFFECTS	COMMENTS
busulfan (Myleran)	PO, INJ	leukemia	*Most common* – NVD, stomatitis, myelosuppression* *Rare but serious* – seizures, lung problems, liver problems *Myelosuppression is a reduction in blood cell components (reduction in red blood cells is anemia; white blood cells is leukopenia/neutropenia; platelets is thrombocytopenia). This renders the patient susceptible to infections and bleeding. The development of myelosuppression limits the dose that can be used for many chemotherapy agents. Correct dosing of chemotherapy is absolutely essential to avoid life-threatening toxicity and death.	
carboplatin (Paraplatin)	INJ	ovarian cancer	*Most common* – NV, myelosuppression *Rare but serious* – severe allergic reactions	
chlorambucil (Leukeran)	PO	leukemia, lymphomas	*Most common* – myelosuppression *Rare but serious* – seizures, cancer	
cisplatin (Platinol)	INJ	testicular, ovarian, bladder cancers	*Most common* – NV, myelosuppression *Rare but serious* – kidney problems, hearing problems, severe allergic reactions, peripheral neuropathy	
cyclophosphamide (Cytoxan)	PO, INJ	lymphomas, leukemia, breast, ovarian cancer	*Most common* – NV, stomatitis, hair loss, hemorrhagic cystitis (bladder bleeding), leukopenia *Rare but serious* – heart damage, cancer	
ifosfamide (Ifex)	PO	testicular cancer	*Most common* – NV, myelosuppression, hair loss, hemorrhagic cystitis *Rare but serious* – coma	Use with mesna to lessen hemorrhagic cystitis.
melphalan (Alkeran)	PO, INJ	multiple myeloma, ovarian cancer	*Most common* – NVD, hair loss, myelosuppression *Rare but serious* – severe allergic reactions, cancer	
oxaliplatin (Eloxatin)	INJ	colon, rectal cancer	*Most common* – NVD, neuropathy *Rare but serious* – severe allergic reactions, myelosuppression	

TABLE 4-4 (continued)

Organ-Specific Listing of Commonly Used Medications

Oncolytic Agents (for cancers, both solid tumors and blood cancers) [continued]

Antimetabolites

GENERIC NAME (BRAND NAME)	DOSAGE FORM	COMMON USES	COMMON/SEVERE ADVERSE EFFECTS	COMMENTS
capecitabine (Xeloda)	PO	breast, colorectal cancers	*Most common* – DNV, stomatitis, myelosuppression *Rare but serious* – heart problems, painful swelling of hands and feet	
cytarabine (Cytosar-U)	INJ	leukemia	*Most common* – NVD, myelosuppression, fever, muscle pain *Rare but serious* – liver problems	Abbreviated ARA-C.
5-fluorouracil (Adrucil)	INJ	colon, rectal, breast, stomach, pancreas cancers	*Most common* – NV, stomatitis, myelosuppression *Rare but serious* – angina, visual problems	Abbreviated 5-FU.
gemcitabine (Gemzar)	INJ	pancreatic, lung cancers	*Most common* – myelosuppression, fever, rash	
hydroxyurea (Hydrea)	PO	melanoma, leukemia	*Most common* – myelosuppression, stomatitis *Rare but serious* – kidney problems	
mercaptopurine (Purinethol)	PO	leukemia	*Most common* – myelosuppression *Rare but serious* – liver problems	
methotrexate	PO, INJ	breast, lung cancers, leukemia, rheumatoid arthritis, psoriasis	*Most common* – stomatitis, leukopenia, N, malaise *Rare but serious* – myelosuppression, liver, lung, and heart problems, severe skin reaction	

Antimitotic Agents

docetaxel (Taxotere)	INJ	breast, lung cancers	*Most common* – myelosuppression, rash, NV, edema, hair loss *Rare but serious* – severe fluid retention	Use corticosteroids to lessen fluid retention.
paclitaxel (Taxol)	INJ	ovarian, breast, lung cancers	*Most common* – myelosuppression, peripheral neuropathy, NVD *Rare but serious* – severe allergic reactions, heart problems	
vinblastine (Velban)	INJ	lymphoma	*Most common* – leukopenia, hair loss, NV *Rare but serious* – breathing problems	Intrathecal administration (around the spine) is usually fatal.
vincristine (Oncovin)	INJ	leukemia, lymphoma	*Most common* – hair loss, C, peripheral neuropathy *Rare but serious* – nerve damage, breathing problems	
vinorelbine (Navelbine)	INJ	lung cancer	*Most common* – myelosuppression, fatigue, CN *Rare but serious* – lung problems	

TABLE 4-4 (continued)

Organ-Specific Listing of Commonly Used Medications

Oncolytic Agents (for cancers, both solid tumors and blood cancers) [continued]

Topoisomerase Inhibitors

GENERIC NAME (BRAND NAME)	DOSAGE FORM	COMMON USES	COMMON/SEVERE ADVERSE EFFECTS	COMMENTS
etoposide (VePesid)	PO, INJ	testicular, lung cancers	*Most common* – myelosuppression, NV *Rare but serious* – severe allergic reactions	Abbreviated VP-16.
irinotecan (Camptosar)	INJ	colon, rectal cancers	*Most common* – D (can be severe), NV, myelosuppression, hair loss	
topotecan (Hycamtin)	INJ	ovarian, lung cancers	*Most common* – myelosuppression, hair loss, NVDC	

Antibiotics (used as chemotherapy)

GENERIC NAME (BRAND NAME)	DOSAGE FORM	COMMON USES	COMMON/SEVERE ADVERSE EFFECTS	COMMENTS
bleomycin (Blenoxane)	INJ	lymphoma, head/neck, testicular cancers, pleural effusion (fluid in lungs)	*Most common* – hair loss, rash, itching, stomatitis, fever, chills, NV *Rare but serious* – lung damage	
daunorubicin	INJ	leukemia	*Most common* – myelosuppression, hair loss, NV, red-colored urine *Rare but serious* – heart damage (related to total dose)	
doxorubicin (Adriamycin)	INJ	leukemia, breast, ovarian, bladder, thyroid cancers, lymphoma	*Most common* – myelosuppression, NV, stomatitis, red-colored urine, hair loss *Rare but serious* – heart damage (related to total dose)	
epirubicin (Ellence)	INJ	breast cancer	*Most common* – hair, loss, myelosuppression, NV, stomatitis, red-colored urine, cessation of menstrual cycles *Rare but serious* – heart damage (related to total dose), leukemia	
idarubicin (Idamycin)	INJ	leukemia	*Most common* – NVD, myelosuppression, hair loss, stomatitis *Rare but serious* – heart damage	
mitoxantrone (Novantrone)	INJ	prostate cancer, leukemia, multiple sclerosis	*Most common* – myelosuppression, NV, menstrual changes, hair loss, blue-green-colored urine *Rare but serious* – heart damage (related to total dose), leukemia	

TABLE 4-4 (continued)

Organ-Specific Listing of Commonly Used Medications

Oncolytic Agents (for cancers, both solid tumors and blood cancers) [continued]

Hormones (used as chemotherapy)

GENERIC NAME (BRAND NAME)	DOSAGE FORM	COMMON USES	COMMON/SEVERE ADVERSE EFFECTS	COMMENTS
anastrozole (Arimidex)	PO	breast cancer	*Most common* – weight gain, flushing	
bicalutamide (Casodex)	PO	prostate cancer	*Most common* – hot flushes, breast enlargement/pain in men, C *Rare but serious* – liver problems	
exemestane (Aromasin)	PO	breast cancer	*Most common* – fatigue, hot flushes, N	
letrozole (Femara)	PO	breast cancer	*Most common* – bone pain, hot flushes, N, back pain	
leuprolide (Lupron)	INJ, implant	prostate cancer, endometriosis	*Most common* – hot flushes, cessation of menstruation	
megestrol (Megace)	PO	breast, endometrial cancers	*Most common* – weight gain *Rare but serious* – blood clots	
tamoxifen (Nolvadex)	PO	breast cancer	*Most common* – hot flushes *Rare but serious* – blood clots, uterine cancer, eye problems	

Monoclonal Antibodies

GENERIC NAME (BRAND NAME)	DOSAGE FORM	COMMON USES	COMMON/SEVERE ADVERSE EFFECTS	COMMENTS
alemtuzumab (Campath)	INJ	leukemia	*Most common* – fever, chill, myelosuppression, NV *Rare but serious* – severe infusion reactions	
bevacizumab (Avastin)	INJ	colon, rectal cancer	*Most common* – nose bleeds, abdominal pain, anorexia, high blood pressure, CD *Rare but serious* – GI perforation, severe bleeding, CHF	
cetuximab (Erbitux)	INJ	colorectal cancer	*Most common* – rash, sun sensitivity, NDC *Rare but serious* – severe infusion reactions, lung problems	
gefitinib (Iressa)	PO	lung cancer	*Most common* – D, rash, acne, N *Rare but serious* – lung problems	
gemtuzumab ozogamicin (Mylotarg)	INJ	leukemia	*Most common* – myelosuppression, NVD, fever *Rare but serious* – severe allergic/infusion reactions, liver problems	
imatinib (Gleevec)	PO	leukemia	*Most common* – edema (fluid retention), DNV, myelosuppression, muscle cramps, sun sensitivity *Rare but serious* – severe rash, liver problems	

TABLE 4-4 (continued)

Organ-Specific Listing of Commonly Used Medications

Oncolytic Agents (for cancers, both solid tumors and blood cancers) [continued]

Monoclonal Antibodies (continued)

GENERIC NAME (BRAND NAME)	DOSAGE FORM	COMMON USES	COMMON/SEVERE ADVERSE EFFECTS	COMMENTS
rituximab (Rituxan)	INJ	lymphoma	*Most common* – N, night sweats, fever, chills, leukopenia *Rare but serious* – fatal infusion reactions, kidney problems, severe rash, heart problems	
trastuzumab (Herceptin)	INJ	breast cancer	*Most common* – DN, fever, chills *Rare but serious* – CHF, severe infusion reactions	

Hematopoietic Agents (treat myelosuppression caused by chemotherapy)

GENERIC NAME (BRAND NAME)	DOSAGE FORM	COMMON USES	COMMON/SEVERE ADVERSE EFFECTS	COMMENTS
darbepoetin alfa (Aranesp)	INJ	anemia	*Most common* – elevated blood pressure	
epoetin alfa (Epogen)	INJ	anemia	*Most common* – elevated blood pressure	
filgrastim (Neupogen)	INJ	neutropenia	*Rare but serious* – severe allergic reactions	

Dermatologic Agents (for the skin)

Anti-Infective Agents (Antibiotics, Antifungal, and Antiviral Drugs)

GENERIC NAME (BRAND NAME)	DOSAGE FORM	COMMON USES	COMMON/SEVERE ADVERSE EFFECTS	COMMENTS
acyclovir (Zovirax)	TOP	herpes genitalis, cold sores	*Most common* – burning, stinging	
clotrimazole (Lotrimin)	TOP	athlete's foot, jock itch, other mild fungal infections	*Most common* – redness, stinging	Some forms available OTC.
mupirocin (Bactroban)	TOP	impetigo, bacterial infections	*Most common* – burning, stinging	
polymyxin B/ neomycin/bacitracin (Neosporin)	TOP	prevent bacterial infection after minor injury	*Most common* – allergic reaction	Available OTC.
terbinafine (Lamisil)	TOP	athlete's foot, jock itch, other fungal infections	*Most common* – irritation, burning	
tolnaftate (Tinactin)	TOP	athlete's foot, jock itch, other mild fungal infections	*Most common* – irritation	Available OTC.

TABLE 4-4 (continued)

Organ-Specific Listing of Commonly Used Medications

Dermatologic Agents (for the skin) [continued]

Topical Corticosteroids

GENERIC NAME (BRAND NAME)	DOSAGE FORM	COMMON USES	COMMON/SEVERE ADVERSE EFFECTS	COMMENTS
betamethasone (example: Diprolene, Valisone)	TOP	inflammation and itching	*Most common* – burning, irritation	
hydrocortisone (example: Hytone)	TOP	↓	↓	Some forms available OTC.
triamcinolone (example: Kenalog)	TOP			

Other Dermatological Agents

capsaicin (Zostrix)	TOP	pain (of conditions such as arthritis and shingles)	*Most common* – significant burning	Available OTC.
isotretinoin (Accutane)	PO	severe acne	*Most common* – dry skin, dry eyes *Rare but serious* –depression, visual problems	Contraindicated in pregnancy.
minoxidil (Rogaine)	TOP	hair growth in men	*Most common* – local irritation *Rare but serious* – fast heart rate, dizziness, blood pressure changes	Available OTC.
pimecrolimus (Elidel)	TOP	dermatitis	*Most common* – burning	

Nutritional Agents (vitamins, nutritional aids and supplements)

calcium	PO, INJ	hypocalcemia (osteoporosis)	*Most common* – C *Rare but serious* – hypercalcemia, heart problems (IV administration)	
iron	PO, INJ	iron-deficiency anemia	*Most common* – N *Rare but serious* – iron overload, severe allergic reactions (IV or IM administration)	Overdose dangerous for young children.
potassium supplements (example: K-Dur)	PO, INJ	hypokalemia (potassium deficiency)	*Most common* – DN *Rare but serious* – hyperkalemia	IV administration can be dangerous and requires heart monitoring.

TABLE 4-4 (continued)

Organ-Specific Listing of Commonly Used Medications

Abbreviations used:

APAP = acetaminophen (Tylenol)

CHF = congestive heart failure

HCTZ = hydrochlorothiazide

NSAID = nonsteroidal anti-inflammatory drug; used for relief of pain and inflammation

OCD = obsessive-compulsive disorder

OTC = over the counter (nonprescription)

EPS = Extrapyramidal symptoms (dyskinesia [abnormal involuntary movements, also called tardive dyskinesia], dystonias [muscle spasms], akathisia [feeling of a need to move around], akinesia [decreased motor activity], and pseudoparkinsonism [drug-induced effects that resemble Parkinson's disease, including decreased motor activity, tremor and pill-rolling motion, cogwheel rigidity in which patients' limbs jerk when moved, and postural problems]).

AC = Anticholinergic side effects (dry mouth, blurred vision, and urinary retention)

OH = Orthostatic hypotension (low blood pressure upon standing up, especially from a lying position, causing the person to feel dizzy or fall

PUD = Peptic ulcer disease (can be in the stomach [gastric] or first part of the small intestine [duodenal])

GERD = Gastroesophageal reflux disease

HTN = Hypertension (high blood pressure)

MI = Myocardial infarction (heart attack)

AF = Atrial fibrillation

PSVT = Paroxysmal supraventricular tachycardia

PO = oral

INJ = injection (could be intravenous, intramuscular, subcutaneous)

Supp = suppository

TOP = topical (example: cream, ointment, patch)

DVT = deep venous thrombosis (blood clot in leg)

PE = pulmonary embolism (blood clot in lung)

UTI = urinary tract infection

Adverse effects abbreviations:

N = Nausea

V = Vomiting

D = Diarrhea

C = Constipation

HA = Headache

GI = Gastrointestinal

alone, and that the cost of DRPs among ambulatory patients (not in hospitals or nursing homes) was determined several years ago to be $177 billion per year in the United States; the current figure is no doubt much higher, given recent rates of inflation of health care costs. If true, these numbers mean that DRPs are one of the leading causes of death, exceeded only by conditions such as cancer and heart problems. Further, for every dollar spent on drugs in ambulatory patients, another dollar or more is spent in health care resources for DRPs. Pharmacists pushed the federal and state governments to fund programs through which they can turn their attention to preventing and resolving DRPs, and this resulted in implementation of a medication therapy management provision in the Medicare Part D benefit mentioned in Chapter 3. As these programs are implemented, pharmacy technicians will become even more important in the process of preparing prescriptions for dispensing, so that pharmacists can apply their skills to DRPs. In addition, observant technicians can point out obvious errors to the pharmacist.

TABLE 4-5

Drug-Related Problems

Some situations in which drugs can cause unexpected harm include:

- Some DRPs, such as *adverse drug reactions,* while unwanted, are expected to occur in a portion of patients on a given drug, as extensions of its desired effects.

- Sometimes patients react to a drug, as in an allergy to the agent. Again, although unexpected in a given patient, we recognize that a certain percentage of patients will exhibit such allergic reactions. In both this example and the previous one, the relative benefits of using the drug are believed to outweigh the inherent risks, thus justifying its use in people.

- Errors can be made in the *prescribing process.* Physicians may misdiagnose a condition, or they may write a prescription for the wrong agent, dose, strength, route of administration, or duration of therapy. One of the main reasons pharmacists instead of physicians dispense prescriptions is so that the pharmacist can catch errors made by the physician.

- Errors can be made in the *dispensing process* at the pharmacy. A major focus during dispensing is summarized this way: "Your job in dispensing is to make sure that the right drug gets to the right patient at the right time, in the right strength, in the right quantity, and in the right dosage form." When any of these details is wrong, an error has occurred; when a patient is injured by the error, a DRP has occurred.

- Finally, the patient, nurse, or other caregiver may make mistakes in taking the drug or giving the drug to the patient. There have been cases of husbands taking their wives' birth-control pills, of patients taking topical or rectal agents by mouth, of patients not realizing when a drug is causing a serious or life-threatening side effect, and of patients not taking their medicines as directed, even with drugs for life-threatening diseases such as heart problems or AIDS. These errors point to the need for education of the patient and caregiver so that they are informed participants in the drug therapy process.

Drug Interactions

It is the duty of the pharmacist, with the aid of the technician, to screen for and minimize drug interactions.

Medications sometimes "interact" with each other such that the anticipated effect of the drug does not occur or adverse reactions are produced. There are many causes of drug interactions and some drugs are more likely to cause interactions than other drugs. An interaction can occur when one drug prevents the absorption of another. For example, many antacids should not be taken with quinolone antibiotics because the elements in the antacids can bind the quinolone and prevent its absorption, resulting in lack of antibiotic effect.

Most drug interactions involve interference with or changes in drug metabolism in the liver. Recall that the liver metabolizes many drugs by a group of enzymes called the cytochrome P450 enzymes, including CYP 3A4 and CYP 2C9. These isoenzymes can be affected by certain drugs to speed up (induce) or slow down (inhibit) the actions of other drugs. For example, erythromycin is a known inhibitor of CYP 3A4. Carbamazepine, an antiseizure or antiepileptic medication, is metabolized by this pathway. If these drugs are taken together, erythromycin can be expected to slow the metabolism of carbamazepine and thereby increase the blood levels of carbamazepine and possibly cause symptoms of toxicity.

Food and herbal remedies can also interact with drugs. It is the duty of the pharmacist, with the aid of the technician, to screen for and minimize drug interactions.

While computer systems used in pharmacies today help to catch drug interactions, professional judgment often comes into play. For example, if the interaction is not anticipated to cause a clinically significant problem and the prescribed drug is really needed for the patient, the pharmacist may decide to proceed with dispensing.

Conclusion

With a background in calculations, terminology, abbreviations, pharmacy law, and now the medications themselves, you are ready to proceed to the true heart of this book: the preparation of prescriptions for dispensing. Let's go to Chapter 5!

For More Information

If you are preparing for the Pharmacy Technician Certification Examination and feel that you need more information about the topics discussed in this chapter, consider studying this source of additional information:

- DiPiro JT, Talbert RL, Yee GC, et al., eds. *Pharmacotherapy: A Pathophysiologic Approach.* 6th ed. New York: McGraw-Hill Publishers; 2005. (*Editor's note: The 7th edition of this text is scheduled to be published in early 2008.*)

References

1. Seeley RR, Stephens TD, Tate P. *Essentials of Anatomy and Physiology.* 3rd ed. St. Louis, MO: Mosby-Year Book, Inc.; 1999: Table 2.1.

2. Emsley J. *The Elements.* 3rd ed. Oxford, U.K.: Clarendon Press; 1998. Accessed at http://web2.airmail.net/uthman/elements_of_body.html, September 5, 2006.

3. Anonymous. Periodic table (large version). Wikipedia: The Free Encyclopedia; 2006.

4. Tortora GJ, Grabowski SR. *Principles of Anatomy and Physiology. Volume 3, Control Systems of the Human Body.* 10th ed. New York: John Wiley & Sons; 2003.

PART II

Prescription Dispensing

CHAPTER FIVE

What Happens When a Prescription Is Processed

This chapter is in all respects the heart of the book. Most technicians spend the majority of their time preparing drugs for dispensing by the pharmacist. Chapter 5 covers in detail what happens from the time a prescription is presented until the drug is delivered to the patient.

Introduction

A prescription usually refers to an order for a drug for an ambulatory patient.

Technicians generally spend most of their time preparing drugs for dispensing by the pharmacist. Chapter 5 describes in detail the process of receiving, checking, preparing, and delivering a prescription or medication order.

A prescription usually refers to an order for a drug for an ambulatory patient. That is, the patient (or his or her representative) presents the prescription (see Figure 5-1) to the pharmacy, and the drug product is in turn delivered to the patient. In hospital, nursing home, and other institutional pharmacies, physician orders contain requests for medications called "medication orders" (see Figure 5-2). Ambulatory patients require more pharmacy services than most institutionalized patients, because they need to know exactly how to take their medications, what each medication is for, and which side effects to watch for. Therefore, we will focus in this chapter on the "prescription" process rather than the "medication order" process. However, if you are working in an institutional pharmacy, you should still find the information to be very pertinent, and differences will be noted when appropriate.

FIGURE 5-1

Example of a prescription.

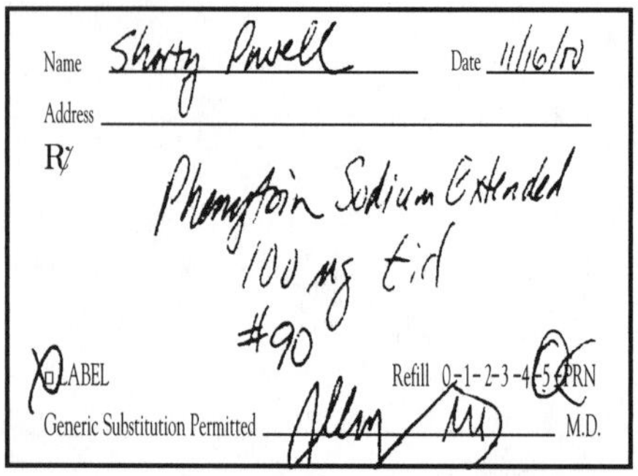

Parts of a Prescription

The parts of a prescription are described in Table 5-1.

Physician order sheets, used in hospitals and other institutions, contain medication orders similar to prescriptions. Order sheets are usually triplicate forms used by physicians and other health professionals to convey a variety of instructions for patients. As shown in Figure 5-2, orders may be from various professionals in an institution, including nurses; pharmacists; respiratory, physical, or occupational therapists; or even social workers. When physician order sheets arrive in the pharmacy, the pharmacist or technician must review them carefully to identify the drug orders on each page.

Because the hospital or institution already has information about patients and prescribers on file, medication orders may not have all of the information usually contained in a prescription as listed in Table 5-1. Additionally, in the institutional setting, orders for Schedule II substances do not have to be separated and stored any differently from other medication orders, as nurses keep those medications in a locked cabinet or automated device on the patient care unit.

When information is missing from prescriptions or medication orders, you may need to talk with the patient, pharmacist, or prescriber.

FIGURE 5-2

Example of a medication order.

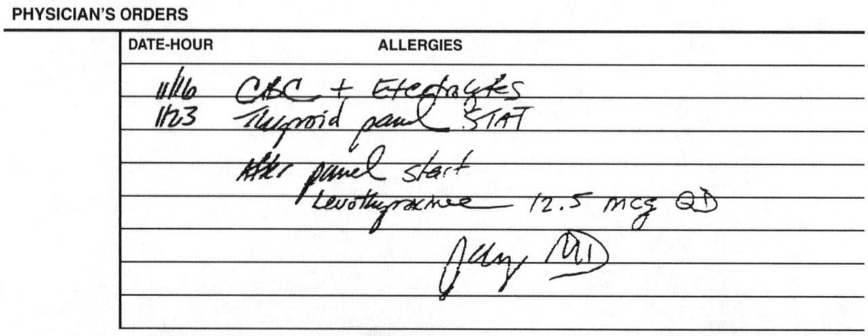

Obtaining Information from Patients and Professionals

When information is missing from prescriptions or medication orders, you may need to talk with the patient, pharmacist, or prescriber. While Chapter 8 will discuss communication strategies with patients in more detail, a few general communications points are appropriate to present now.

Any contact you as a technician have with the patient or prescriber should be within the guidelines established by your institution, pharmacy, or supervising pharmacist. Patients have a right to privacy with respect to their health, and you must take care as to when and how you talk with them. In most pharmacies, technicians assist in clarifying the spelling of patients' names or getting their addresses, but be sure you know what other information you are responsible for obtaining.

Similarly, contact you have with the prescriber should be within the guidelines of your pharmacy or employer. Pharmacists may prefer—or even be required by law—to contact the prescriber directly about unclear critical information, such as the name of the drug or instructions on how to use it, whether a dose is correct, or whether the patient is allergic to a drug. In particular, if you think a prescription may be forged, be certain to work with the pharmacist in contacting the prescriber to verify it (see Chapter 3 for more information about forged prescriptions).

Most pharmacies regularly record patients' ages and weights because this information is sometimes needed in checking medication doses. In an institution, pharmacists likely obtain this information from patients' medical records or computer profiles. However, such sensitive information may not be so readily available in a community pharmacy. The best method of asking about age and weight is as a part of a written questionnaire that community pharmacists often have patients complete when they have their first prescription filled. If you need to ask patients for their ages and weights, be sure that you do so in a quiet and respectful manner. You never want to offend a patient or embarrass someone in front of their friends and neighbors.

Another type of information you may need to collect concerns the patient's insurance or health coverage. Again, because this is confidential information, take care to obtain it in an appropriate manner. Errors in the beneficiaries' names, policy numbers, and other information can cause claims to be rejected, so take care to record this information carefully. To be sure you can hear the patient, insurance and health coverage information is best collected in a quiet area.

Processing the Prescription

Once you have obtained all necessary information and you are satisfied that the prescription is valid, you are ready to prepare the medication for the patient. The act of transferring a medication to the patient is central to the entire practice of pharmacy. It is that act for which the entire system and profession exist. Your assistance in this process constitutes a heavy responsibility that you must take very seriously.

An old adage in pharmacy is that, in dispensing prescriptions, you must get the right drug in the right dosage form to the right patient at the right time, labeled with the right directions and other instructions. Let's look at the process of making sure all these things happen correctly.

TABLE 5-1

Parts of a Prescription

As shown in Figure 5-1, a prescription has the following parts:

- Patient name, and, for controlled substances, a full address.
- Date the prescriber wrote the prescription. This is especially important because state laws often specify that prescriptions are valid for only 1 year after they are written.
- Rx symbol—standing for the Latin verb "recipe," meaning "you take."
- Name of the medication (the "inscription"). Prescribers may use either generic or brand names. In the case of compounded prescriptions, the prescriber may list several ingredients that the pharmacist is to mix together.
- Directions to the pharmacist on what to dispense (the "subscription"). This usually consists of a number of tablets or capsules, a volume of a liquid, or one or more prepackaged medications from a manufacturer.
- Directions on how the medication is to be used (the "sig," which is short for "signa," Latin for "write"). Prescribers use abbreviations, such as those presented in Chapter 2, to convey to the pharmacist how the patient should take the medication.
- Refills, special labeling, or other instructions. Prescriptions may not be refilled without the prescriber's permission. Per federal law, prescriptions for Schedule II controlled substances cannot be refilled at all. Prescriptions for Schedule III through V substances may be refilled, with the prescriber's permission, up to five times over the 6-month period beginning on the day the prescription is written, not dispensed.
- Prescriber's signature and, for controlled substances, the DEA number (see Chapter 3).

FIGURE 5-3

Any contact you as a technician have with the patient or prescriber should be within the guidelines established by your institution, pharmacy, or supervising pharmacist.

Understanding Generic and Brand Names

Every bit of information on a prescription is important, but certainly the most important element is the name of the drug or drug product. As mentioned in Chapter 4, drugs may be prescribed by their generic and brand names. The generic name is the common name assigned to that chemical compound by the US Adopted Names Council; it may be used by any company that markets the drug. The brand name is a trademarked reference to the drug that only one company is entitled to use. This company is usually the innovator, or original creator, of that drug. Until its patent on the drug expires, the innovator is the only company entitled to market the drug. When a drug is available from only one company, it is called *single-source product*. For example, Prevacid, shown in Figure 5-3, is a single-source product until the innovator's patent expires. When a drug is available from more than one company, it is called a *multisource product*. Notice in Figure 5-4 that all the products have the same generic name, glipizide, but the innovator product also has a trade name, Glucotrol. Occasionally generic products also have a brand name; these are called branded generics, but they are still essentially just generic alternatives to the originator branded product.

When you read a prescription, read the name of the drug (and all other information) very carefully. Many mistakes in pharmacy occur as a result of poor handwriting on the part of physicians or misreading of drug names by pharmacy personnel. If the name of the drug does not fit the directions for use (for instance, wrong number of doses per day or wrong route of administration) or if you are not 100% certain of what the prescriber has written, you or the pharmacist must contact the prescriber to clarify the name of the drug. It is not enough to guess about the drug by asking the patient "what they went to the doctor for."

If a prescription is written for a brand-name drug but other (usually cheaper) generic products are available, you must follow the laws in your state concerning generic substitution (Figure 5-5). In several states, you must inform the patient of the availability of the lower-cost agents and let the patient decide which product he or she wants. If the prescriber has written "Brand Product Necessary" on the prescription or checked a box for "Dispense As Written," you must follow the prescriber's instructions and give the patient the brand-name product. Talk with the pharmacists you work with about how to handle these situations in your pharmacy and your state.

Another situation that affects the drug dispensed occurs with some Medicaid or managed care plans. When patients are covered by third-party payers, like a state Medicaid system or insurance company (as nearly all are these days), the pharmacy is obligated by contract to fill some prescriptions with drugs that are similar to ones a prescriber may request but that are not the same chemically. This is called therapeutic substitution or drug-product selection. Again, talk with your pharmacists about what contracts the pharmacy has and what policies must be followed for patients covered under those plans.

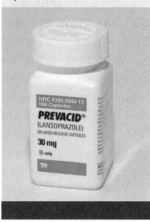

Single-source product.

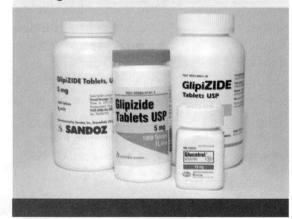

FIGURE 5-4

Multisource products, showing the innovator product (Glucotrol) and generic alternatives.

Preparing the Medication Label

The first step in filling the prescription is preparing the label that will be put on the vial or drug product. Because this is what the patient will read to know how to use the medication, the label must be clear in its instructions, prepared neatly, and affixed firmly to the final prescription packaging.

Under the pharmacy laws of your state, certain information must be put on the prescription label. While these laws vary, most states require the information presented in Table 5-2.

Many states also require the name of the medication and the strength dispensed. The brand name should be used only when the product dispensed is the brand-name drug; otherwise, the generic name should be used.

You must read the prescription to learn most of the above information, and you will usually need to interpret the Latin pharmaceutical abbreviations presented in Chapter 2 to do so. If you are not 100% certain of what the prescriber has written or requested, then you must contact him or her for clarification. In addition, if you are not completely sure that you remember what the Latin abbreviations stand for, ask for help from the pharmacist or other technicians.

Almost all pharmacies are now computerized, so the process of preparing the prescription label is generally automated. You must learn the codes that are used in your pharmacy's software to make the correct directions print out on the label. Because small errors in putting these codes into the computer can cause serious mistakes on the label, be sure to read the label after it prints out to be certain that the directions are correct.

In addition, you will need to be able to produce labels when the computer system is down. This usually involves using a typewriter and requires you to remember the proper information that goes on prescription labels.

Obtaining and Checking Medications

Once you determine the drug product the prescriber has requested, you must retrieve it from the storage area and bring it back to the product-preparation area. Before you get the product, you must know the name of the drug, the strength of the drug (for example, 25 mg or 50 mg), the dosage form requested (for example, tablets, liquids, eye drops, or ear drops), and the quantity you need. If you cannot remember these four details, then take the written prescription or the printed labels with you to retrieve the product.

During the dispensing process, 100% accuracy is needed. Most pharmacists strive to achieve this level of perfection by checking the prescription three times: once when they get the product from the shelf, once when they begin to measure the product, and once after they affix the prescription label to the vial.

In the process of getting products from the storage shelves or bins, many mistakes occur when pharmacy personnel rely on the color of a package or the shape of a box rather than reading the name of the drug product. Be certain you have pulled the right product to begin with, and prevent medication errors (Figure 5-6).

TABLE 5-2

The Prescription Label

Information that must be on the prescription label includes:

- Pharmacy name and address
- A sequential number that enables the pharmacy to retrieve the prescription from the files
- Patient's name
- Date the prescription was filled
- Prescriber's name
- Directions for use of the medication
- The federal legend: "Caution: Federal law prohibits transfer of this drug to any person other than the patient for whom it was prescribed."

FIGURE 5-5

Three different levothyroxine products.

Depending on state laws, prescriber directions, patient preferences, and facts about bioequivalence as determined by the U.S. Food and Drug Administration, the pharmacist may or may not want to substitute a generic alternative for the prescribed brand of medication.

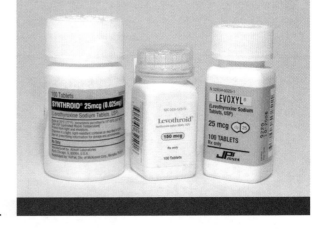

Pharmacy technician checking that she is pulling the correct product.

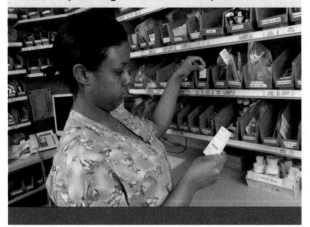

As the number of approved drugs has exploded over the past half century, the process of coming up with unique generic and brand names has become more and more difficult. As a result, many names are similar in the way they are spelled and/or pronounced. To avoid medication errors that result from look-alike names, pharmaceutical companies have begun putting the unique parts of generic names in upper case letters, as shown in Figure 5-7. This helps to avoid medication errors caused when someone retrieves the wrong bottle of medication from pharmacy shelves or storage areas.

The correct dosage form is just as important as the right drug. For instance, if you accidentally give a patient ear drops and they are placed in the eyes, the patient could suffer permanent eyesight damage. Be certain that you know what the prescriber is asking for and that you have pulled the right product, and also whether it's a cream or ointment, syrup or elixir, tablet or capsule, or a short- or long-acting product (Figure 5-8).

Finally, the right strength is also critical. Some drugs—such as levothyroxine (Figure 5-9)—have narrow therapeutic indexes, meaning that the right dose in one patient may be toxic in the next patient. Again, be sure that you have retrieved the exact strength the prescriber is asking for, whether it's 100 µg or 100 mg, 0.1 mg or 1 mg, 1% or 10%, or 125 mg/5 mL or 250 mg/5 mL.

And, of course, you need to get enough product for the prescription, whether it's for 10 tablets or 100 capsules, 1 oz or 2 L, or 1 inhaler or 20 suppositories. Otherwise, you will waste valuable time in going back for more—and you may accidentally pull the wrong package when you go back hurriedly or when you get frustrated.

During the dispensing process, 100% accuracy is needed.

Measuring Drug Products

Measuring solid oral drug products is generally fairly simple—for tablets and capsules, you just need to count out the appropriate number. For this purpose, most pharmacies have counting trays (Figure 5-10), and many have automated counting devices that can

Look-alike generic names with unique portions of names in upper case letters.

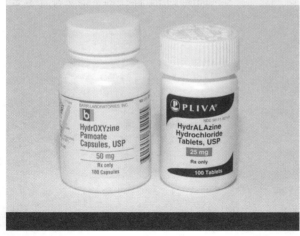

Example of a drug available in several dosage forms and formulations.

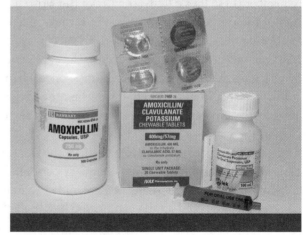

FIGURE 5-9

Levothyroxine must be dosed very carefully, and several strengths are available so that prescribers can titrate doses to the exact needs of the patient.

The correct dosage form is just as important as the right drug.

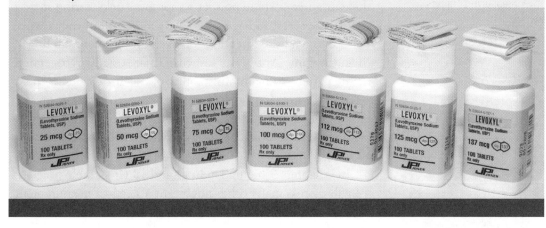

save you time (Figure 5-11). Be sure that these devices are kept clean; otherwise one patient's drugs can contaminate the next patient's drugs. In the case of agents that many people are allergic to, like penicillin, this amount of contamination has sometimes been associated with serious reactions.

When measuring liquids, you need clean graduated cylinders or other appropriate equipment (Figure 5-12). Take a graduated cylinder and put some water in it. Notice how the liquid curves, with the higher edges on the sides and the lower level in the middle. When reading the amount of liquid in any measuring device, you always read at the bottom of this curve, which is called the *meniscus*.

Many antibiotics come from the manufacturer as powders in a bottle (see bottle of amoxicillin on the right side of Figure 5-8 for

FIGURE 5-11

Automated tablet counters.
Automated tablet counters are used in many pharmacies to quickly and accurately obtain the needed numbers of tablets and capsules for individual patient prescriptions.

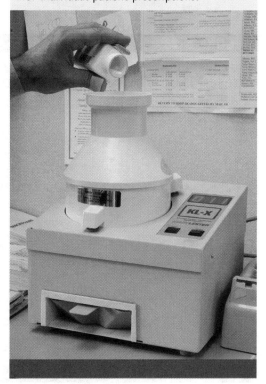

FIGURE 5-10

Counting trays.
Counting trays, which have come to symbolize pharmacy in recent years, are used to obtain the correct numbers of tablets or capsules.

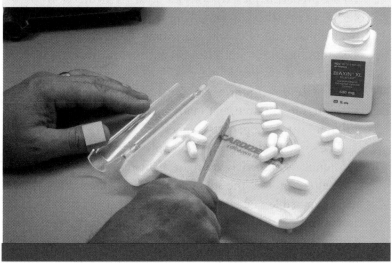

FIGURE 5-12

Equipment for measuring liquids.

Graduated cylinders, funnels, beakers, and mortars and pestles are used during prescription filling in the pharmacy for tasks such as measuring liquids and grinding solids into powders.

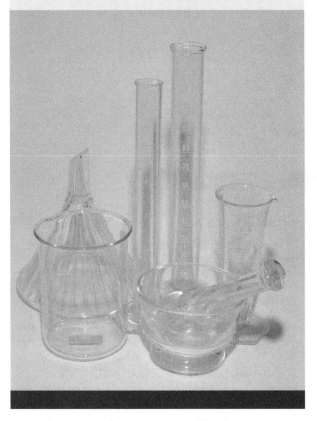

FIGURE 5-13

Prescription vials used for solid oral dosage forms (tablets and capsules).

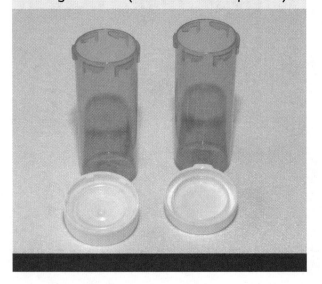

example). You must add the appropriate amount of water (usually distilled water) to the bottle and shake it well to prepare a suspension of the antibiotic. Also check the bottom of the container—where powder sometimes sticks during storage—to be sure you have completely mixed all of the powder. Be sure to read the directions on each antibiotic and follow them carefully. Antibiotic suspensions are usually refrigerated by the patient to maintain stability of the antibiotic for the 10 or so days of drug administration. Also, the patient must understand the importance of shaking the bottle immediately before pouring a dose. Be clear on whether the bottle must be refrigerated.

In Chapters 9 (compounding) and 10 (injectable drugs), we will discuss many other important aspects of measurement of drugs and drug products, including the use of scales and syringes.

Packaging the Prescription and Affixing the Label

Once the label is prepared and the drug product has been counted or measured, you are ready to place the drug in the actual container the patient will receive. Drugs must be stored in tight containers so that the moisture and oxygen in the air will not cause them to degrade, or lose their effectiveness, before the patient finishes taking the prescription. For this reason, special prescription vials are used. These vials—usually brown—limit the amount of light that the drug product is exposed to, because some drugs can be degraded by light (Figures 5-13 and 5-14).

In the pharmacy where you work, appropriate prescription vials for solid oral dosage forms will be provided for your use. Try to use the smallest possible vial that will hold the tablets or capsules, which limits the amount of air in the vial.

Under federal law, you must use vials with child-resistant containers unless the patient requests easy-open tops. When you are preparing prescriptions for arthritis medications or for older patients who are unlikely to have children at home, ask them which kind of closure they want. If they ask for easy-open tops, be sure to tell them to put their medicines in a safe place when their grandchildren or other young visitors are around. Child-resistant containers have greatly reduced poisonings in children, but many incidents still occur when children visit grandparents' homes.

The same guiding principles apply to prescription vials for oral liquids. These vials are tight, light-resistant containers that help to protect the stability of drug products. Use the smallest possible vial, and use vials with child-resistant closures unless the patient asks for easy-open containers. When measuring the liquid in these vials, the meniscus should be at the correct line on the side of the vial.

FIGURE 5-14

Prescription bottle used for oral liquid dosage forms (syrups, elixirs, suspensions, and solutions).

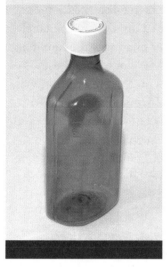

FIGURE 5-15

Unit-of-use packaging is increasingly available from pharmaceutical companies.

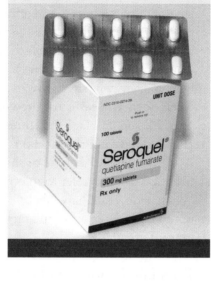

FIGURE 5-16

Bubble Packaging. Bubble packaging is used for preparing individual patient's medications for administration in nursing homes or to help patients at home remember which drugs to take at specific times of the day.

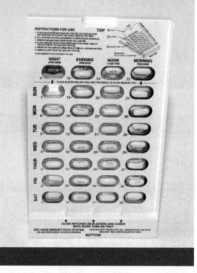

Many drug products today come in packages that are appropriate for dispensing directly to the patient. An example of such packaging is *oral contraceptives* (birth control pills), which come in 21- or 28-day supplies with the days of the week or numbers marked so that the patient can remember if she has taken her medicine. This is called *unit-of-use packaging* because it is prepared by the manufacturer in the most commonly dispensed unit. It is used increasingly for various types of prescription drugs (Figure 5-15), and pharmacies also prepare individualized packaging for use in nursing homes and to help patients at home remember what medicines to take at which times of day (Figure 5-16).

Many drug products today come in packages that are appropriate for dispensing directly to the patient.

FIGURE 5-17

Affixing the prescription label to the vial.

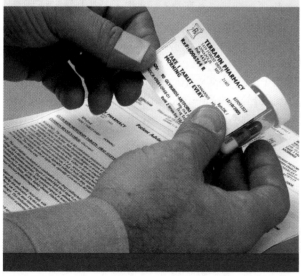

Once you have put the prescription product in the appropriate container, you are ready to affix the prescription label (Figure 5-17). Either before or after you do, stop for a moment and check everything: the drug product, the directions on the label, even the names of the patient and prescriber. Be sure that you have everything correct before you pass the prescription on to the pharmacist for the final check.

For unit-of-use packages, the prescription label will be placed somewhere on the container.

FIGURE 5-18

Adding auxiliary labels to the prescription vial.

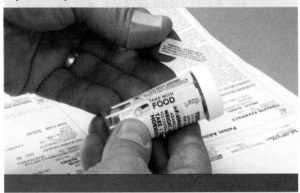

FIGURE 5-19

Pharmacist counseling patient.

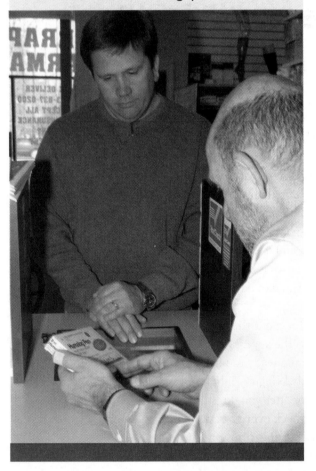

Some pharmacists prefer to place products such as eye or ear drops in larger bottles so that the full prescription label can be affixed. In addition, bottles of nitroglycerin tablets are too small for a label, but the tablets must be kept in the original container to maintain product stability. Put the original container inside a larger prescription vial, and affix the label to the larger vial.

Most pharmacies also put auxiliary labels on prescription vials (Figure 5-18), although these are being displaced somewhat by special messages that are printed directly on the label by pharmacy computer software. If your pharmacy uses auxiliary labels, such as "May cause drowsiness" or "For external use only," be sure to place the correct ones on the prescription vial after you have put the label on. The pharmacist will need to teach you which labels he or she wants put on which drug products. You can also refer to information such as that in Table 4-4. When adding auxiliary labels to the prescription vial, take care not to cover any part of the prescription label or other important information.

Providing Information to Patients

As recently as the mid-1900s, pharmacists were forbidden under both law and ethical standards to tell patients the identity of medicines that were being dispensed. Any questions about the drug or what it was used for were to be referred to the prescriber.

Today, pharmacists are responsible not only for telling patients what the medications are and what they are used for (Figure 5-19), but also for undertaking a full range of patient-education activities. To assist in this role, nearly all prescriptions are dispensed with written information detailing what the drug is, how it works, and what side effects the patient should watch for. This information sometimes prints out of the computer system with the label, while other times it comes in the package with the drug product. In addition, some pharmacies purchase leaflets about commonly dispensed drugs to give to patients.

When you prepare the prescription, place any necessary information with the completed prescription so that it can be given to the patient and, many times, explained to the patient by the pharmacist. This information will generally reinforce the auxiliary labels that you have put on the container with the prescription label.

Performing the Final Check

When you are sure that you have put the right drug in the right strength and dosage form in the right container for the right patient, you are ready to send the prescription to the pharmacist for a final check (Figure 5-20). With the availability of pharmacy computer systems and devices such as scanners, this check is often now linked to the computer system. The pharmacist can check your work by reviewing on the computer screen a scanned copy of the written prescription, a picture of the correct tablet or capsule, and the instructions you entered into the computer.

Using older systems, the pharmacist can check the actual written prescription, the label you prepared, and which bottle you used to obtain the medication. Once the pharmacist is satisfied that everything is correct, he or she will dispense (or authorize the transfer of) the prescription to the patient. Under pharmacy laws of all states, this act of dispensing the medication must be performed by a registered pharmacist.

Chapter 14, Quality Assurance and Control, provides more specific information about the need for accuracy in prescription dispensing.

Conclusion

In this chapter, we have considered in a somewhat simplistic manner the process of preparing a prescription for dispensing to the patient. However, two factors make this process more complicated than we have discussed directly. One is the role the pharmacist plays in making sure that the drug the prescriber has requested is in reality the best choice for a specific patient. The other, which has been mentioned, is the use of pharmacy computer systems and other types of automation in the process of drug dispensing and distribution.

These two topics are covered in detail in the next two chapters. Let's see what they're about!

For More Information

If you are preparing for the Pharmacy Technician Certification Examination and feel that you need more information about the topics discussed in this chapter, consider studying these sources of additional information, both available in the APhA's pharmacist.com Store:

- Snipe K. Technician responsibilities in the community pharmacy. In: *The Pharmacy Technician Skills-Building Manual.* Washington, D.C.: American Pharmacists Association; 2007: 9–22.
- Moss Marks S, Hopkins WA Jr. *Pharmacy Technician Certification Quick-Study Guide.* 3rd edition. Washington, D.C.: American Pharmacists Association; 2006.

When you are sure that you have put the right drug in the right strength and dosage form in the right container for the right patient, you are ready to send the prescription to the pharmacist for a final check.

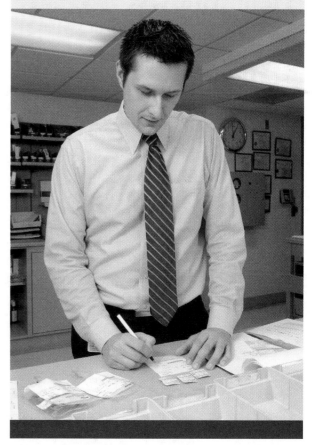

FIGURE 5-20

Hospital pharmacist performing final check.

CHAPTER SIX

Assisting with Medication Therapy Management Services

Chapter 6 describes the pharmacist's emphasis on medication therapy management services and ways that technicians assist in data collection, patient interviews, and data entry and analysis during such pharmaceutical care activities.

Introduction

The assistance pharmacy technicians provide with the dispensing aspect of pharmacy practice has been instrumental in allowing pharmacists to expand into more clinical roles. But technicians are also helping with many of the tasks associated with these new and emerging clinical functions. Now called medication therapy management or pharmaceutical care, the new responsibilities are important for you to both understand and participate in.

Emergence of Pharmaceutical Care

As the pharmaceutical industry emerged and developed in the late 19th and 20th centuries, manufacturers developed technology that enabled mass production of ready-to-dispense tablets, capsules, suppositories, liquids, and injectables. Prescriptions, which previously were very individualized, became so standardized that pharmaceutical companies gave physicians preprinted prescription pads complete with drug name, quantity to dispense, and directions. The only individualization was the patient's name and the prescription number. This changed the art of pharmacy compounding into a routine act of dispensing—a sequence derogatorily referred to as counting, pouring, licking, and sticking.

Luckily, this same threatening development—the industrialization of pharmaceutical manufacturing in the first half of the 20th century—also provided the profession of pharmacy with opportunity. As new and more powerful drugs came onto the market, other health professionals came to rely on pharmacists to provide quick, accurate, and unbiased information.

Beginning at first in hospitals, three simultaneous trends served as the basis for what became known as the *clinical pharmacy movement*: (1) drug information, (2) drug distribution, especially decentralized programs in hospitals, and (3) teaching and research programs in pharmacology and biopharmaceutics. These trends accelerated in the 1970s as increasing numbers of pharmacy schools established clinical sites for their faculty members and students and as the American Pharmaceutical (now Pharmacists) Association (APhA) established the Board of Pharmaceutical Specialties to recognize specialties in pharmacy practice (see Chapter 3).

The clinical pharmacy movement continued in the 1980s. The term "pharmacotherapist" was chosen to designate specialists in clinical pharmacy when the Board of Pharmaceutical Specialties recognized this part of practice in 1988. Board-certified pharmacotherapy specialists carry the initials BCPS following their names.

About this time, Charles D. Hepler, a pharmacy educator, began to argue that the clinical pharmacy and pharmacotherapy movement was not the sole answer to pharmacy's problems. At the 1985 Directions for Clinical Practice in Pharmacy conference (commonly called the Hilton Head conference because of its South Carolina site), Hepler expounded on the notion that pharmacists had to do more than just try to control the use of drugs. He preached that pharmacists needed to take responsibility for the care provided to patients through the clinical use of drugs. In 1987, he first applied the term *pharmaceutical care* in describing what he and colleague Linda Strand called these new, self-actualizing roles for pharmacists.

The definition of pharmaceutical care as proposed by Hepler and Strand is shown in Table 6-1. Several trends were reflected in the concept. For many years, health care institutions and organizations had relied on *process criteria* in judging various systems. If a pharmacist used the correct process for filling a prescription, then the results of that process were assumed to be of adequate quality. The pharmaceutical care definition presented more contemporary *outcomes criteria* in the first paragraph. Thus, where a hospital in the past might have been required to have a certain type of drug-distribution system, the hospital became more concerned with medication error rates. Instead of trying to define the process, the outcomes were of primary interest.

TABLE 6-1

Definition of Pharmaceutical Care

Pharmaceutical care is the responsible provision of drug therapy for the purpose of achieving definite outcomes that improve a patient's quality of life. These outcomes are (1) cure of a disease; (2) elimination or reduction of a patient's symptomatology; (3) arresting or slowing of a disease process; and (4) preventing a disease or symptomatology.

Pharmaceutical care involves the process through which a pharmacist cooperates with a patient and other professionals in designing, implementing, and monitoring a therapeutic plan that will produce specific therapeutic outcomes for the patient. This in turn involves three major functions: (1) identifying potential and actual drug-related problems; (2) resolving actual drug-related problems; and (3) preventing potential drug-related problems.

Pharmaceutical care is a necessary element of health care, and should be integrated with other elements. Pharmaceutical care is, however, provided for the direct benefit of the patient, and the pharmacist is responsible directly to the patient for the quality of that care. The fundamental relationship in pharmaceutical care is a mutually beneficial exchange in which the patient grants authority to the provider, and the provider gives competence and commitment (accepts responsibility) to the patient.

The fundamental goals, processes, and relationships of pharmaceutical care exist regardless of practice setting.

Source: Hepler CD, Strand LM. Opportunities and responsibilities in pharmaceutical care. Am J Pharm Educ 1990; 47:543-9.

Within the pharmaceutical care definition, the four outcomes shown in the first paragraph were related to the purposes for which a medication was being administered to a patient.

The team approach was endorsed in the second paragraph, reflecting pharmacy's shared purpose with other health care professions. The kinds of functions a pharmacist would be expected to provide under pharmaceutical care were also identified in that paragraph.

The third paragraph was the key to the concept of pharmaceutical care. The definition established the idea that the pharmacist has a direct relationship with the patient and a direct responsibility to that patient to provide competent pharmaceutical care (as defined in the first two paragraphs). If the pharmacist does not provide services appropriate to those of a profession (value, complexity, and specificity), then Hepler and Strand argued that the pharmacist has broken his or her professional covenant (or promise) with that patient.

Finally, the fourth paragraph stated that the provision of pharmaceutical care should occur anytime and anywhere a pharmacist encounters a patient. Pharmacists practicing in hospitals were perceived at the time to be practicing at a higher level than were most pharmacists in community practice; therefore, Hepler and Strand wanted to make it clear that pharmaceutical care should encompass all parts of the profession. The same principles applied, they argued, whether the patient was lying in an intensive-care unit at a major medical center or asking about a sunburn in a busy seaside chain pharmacy.

The concept of pharmaceutical care struck a responsive chord with many practitioners. It was termed pharmacy's mission for the 1990s, and pharmaceutical care and the quality of care to patients were linked.

The concept of pharmaceutical care struck a responsive chord with many practitioners. It was termed pharmacy's mission for the 1990s, and pharmaceutical care and the quality of care to patients were linked.

MTM: Pharmaceutical Care Sprouts in Community Pharmacies

Over the years, the contributions that pharmacists can make to improving drug therapy have been recognized in federal laws. In 1974 and again in 1987, the federal government ruled that consultant pharmacists must check the medication regimens of nursing home residents each month and ask the physician to address any problems detected during these reviews.

Johnson and Bootman calculated for every dollar spent on medications for ambulatory Americans (those using the medications outside hospitals and nursing homes) another dollar was spent for medication-related problems, including deaths, hospitalizations, physician office visits, and other medications and treatments.

In 1990, Congress passed a law stating that pharmacists must offer counsel to ambulatory Medicaid patients about their medications. This requirement was extended to all patients by many state boards of pharmacy (see Chapter 3). The federal government thus recognized (1) drugs are not always used properly, even when physicians order them, and (2) pharmacists have the knowledge and expertise to help both the physician and the consumer make sure medications are used properly.

In 1995, an important article in the *Archives of Internal Medicine* confirmed and quantified just how extensive were problems related to suboptimal medication use. Johnson and Bootman showed that medications were a serious and substantial cause of problems among Americans, a finding that was later supported by reports from the respected Institute of Medicine. In fact, Johnson and Bootman calculated, for every dollar spent on medications for ambulatory Americans (those using the medications outside hospitals and nursing homes), another dollar was spent for medication-related problems, including deaths, hospitalizations, physician office visits, and other medications and treatments. This figure was updated in the *Journal of the American Pharmaceutical Association* by Ernst and Grizzle in 2001, and it had more than doubled, from $76 billion in the 1995 study to $177 billion.

Recognition of such problems led innovative practitioners and the APhA Foundation to implement several community-based pharmaceutical care projects in the late 1990s. One of the more important efforts began in 1997 when the City of Asheville, N.C., began contracting with local pharmacists to provide pharmaceutical care services to employees and their dependents with diabetes. Joined later by the Mission St. Joseph's Health System in that city, the Asheville Project demonstrated that pharmacists could reduce the overall cost of health care and improve the lives and work productivity of people with diabetes.

The APhA Foundation expanded the demonstration of pharmacists' services with a series of Project ImPACT (Improving Persistence And Compliance with Therapy) and Patient Self-Management Project studies in the late 1990s and early years of the 21st century. Pharmacists—acting as pharmacotherapy experts, educators, and coaches to patients with chronic diseases such as diabetes, hyperlipidemia, asthma, hypertension, coronary artery disease, and depression—helped people make therapeutic lifestyle changes (getting more exercise, stopping smoking, reducing alcohol intake, and losing weight), take their medications as prescribed, avoid or minimize disease, and in general have a better quality of life.

Also during these years, pharmacists were becoming important sources of immunizations for the American people, especially against influenza. By 2005, all but a few states had changed their laws to permit pharmacists to administer immunizations, and one study had demonstrated that states permitting pharmacist vaccination had lower rates of influenza infections than did other states. By 2004, APhA had certified 15,000 pharmacists and student pharmacists in immunization delivery, and immunizations were a recognized catalyst moving pharmacists from dispensing to a focus on direct patient care.

Congress in December 2003 passed the Medicare Prescription Drug, Improvement, and Modernization Act (MMA), creating Part D of the Medicare program (see Chapter 3). As a result of the recognition of medication-related problems and the important roles pharmacists could play in preventing and resolving them, this law created a Medication Therapy Management (MTM) Services benefit for those patients who have several chronic diseases, take multiple medications for those diseases, and have expected annual drug costs above a level that is adjusted annually (for 2006 and 2007, this figure was $4,000).

By recognizing pharmacists as providers under Medicare and establishing a revenue stream, MTM services have the potential to transform the community pharmacy into the health and wellness center that many pharmacists have dreamed of. While the uptake on MTM services was initially slow, many believe that such patient-centered services—rather than the traditional focus on drug preparation—will define the future roles of pharmacists. If true, technicians will need to be proficient in drug-distribution tasks so that pharmacists will be able to spend time with patients without constant interruptions that characterize the drug-preparation and distribution process.

Medication Therapy Management Responsibilities Under Medicare Part D

Pharmacy is now working to incorporate MTM services into everyday practice in a broad variety of settings. Soon after passage of MMA, APhA convened meetings of key pharmacy associations to develop a consensus-wide definition of MTM services. The result is the language shown in Table 6-2.

To fulfill these MTM tasks, pharmacists mostly rely on technicians to spearhead the drug-preparation phase of the dispensing process. In addition, they are calling on technicians to assist with MTM activities, especially in three key areas:

- Collecting and recording information from patients, other health professionals, or medical records
- Measuring and recording clinical indicators in specific patients, including blood pressures, serum glucose levels, and lipids profiles
- Assisting the pharmacist with activities such as administering medications, especially vaccines; fitting medical devices, such as ostomies; and setting up and educating patients about devices, such as infusion pumps

Collecting and Recording Information

Much of the information needed for MTM can easily be collected by pharmacy technicians. As shown in Table 6-3, while some of this information is sensitive personal information such as sexual history, pharmacy technicians routinely assist pharmacists in gathering straightforward facts from patients.

As pharmacists have developed increasingly sophisticated MTM systems and processes, paper forms and computerized entry programs have been developed and marketed. An example of such forms is shown in Figure 6-1. As you assist the pharmacist in data collection, you may be using a printed form or a computer data-entry screen to record the information. Be very careful to record the information accurately and in the correct space, because errors could compromise patient care or result in denial of payment by third-party payers. In addition, as will be discussed further in Chapter 8, take care to protect the confidentiality of the health-related information you learn through your job as a pharmacy technician.

With the information gathered about patients and their health, the pharmacist performs the additional tasks listed in Table 6-2.

Measuring Clinical Indicators

As mentioned above, monitoring is a very important aspect of pharmaceutical care. How patients respond to various medications (as well as nondrug therapies, such as improved diet or exercise) determines whether medication therapy should be continued, stopped, or altered.

Some patients need more attention than others. For instance, a patient with high blood pressure (hypertension) and diabetes is at risk for further problems and needs a great deal of education and monitoring. On the other hand, a young woman whose only medication is oral contraceptives does not necessarily need counseling, education, and monitoring to the

By 2005, all but a few states had changed their laws to permit pharmacists to administer immunizations, and one study had demonstrated that states permitting pharmacist vaccination had lower rates of influenza infections than did other states.

MTM services have the potential to transform the community pharmacy into the health and wellness center that many pharmacists have dreamed of.

TABLE 6-2

Medication Therapy Management Services: Definition and Program Criteria

Medication Therapy Management is a distinct service or group of services that optimize therapeutic outcomes for individual patients. Medication Therapy Management services are independent of, but can occur in conjunction with, the provision of a medication product.

Medication Therapy Management encompasses a broad range of professional activities and responsibilities within the licensed pharmacist's, or other qualified health care provider's, scope of practice. These services include but are not limited to the following, according to the individual needs of the patient:

a. Performing or obtaining necessary assessments of the patient's health status

b. Formulating a medication treatment plan

c. Selecting, initiating, modifying, or administering medication therapy

d. Monitoring and evaluating the patient's response to therapy, including safety and effectiveness

e. Performing a comprehensive medication review to identify, resolve, and prevent medication-related problems, including adverse drug events

f. Documenting the care delivered and communicating essential information to the patient's other primary care providers

g. Providing verbal education and training designed to enhance patient understanding and appropriate use of his/her medications

h. Providing information, support services, and resources designed to enhance patient adherence with his/her therapeutic regimens

i. Coordinating and integrating medication therapy management services within the broader health care management services being provided to the patient

A program that provides coverage for Medication Therapy Management services shall include:

a. Patient-specific and individualized services or sets of services provided directly by a pharmacist to the patient.[a] These services are distinct from formulary development and use, generalized patient education and information activities, and other population-focused quality assurance measures for medication use.

b. Face-to-face interaction between the patient[a] and the pharmacist as the preferred method of delivery. When patient-specific barriers to face-to-face communication exist, patients shall have equal access to appropriate alternative delivery methods. Medication Therapy Management programs shall include structures supporting the establishment and maintenance of the patient–pharmacist relationship.

c. Opportunities for pharmacists and other qualified health care providers to identify patients who should receive Medication Therapy Management services.

d. Payment for Medication Therapy Management services consistent with contemporary provider payment rates that are based on the time, clinical intensity, and resources required to provide services (e.g., Medicare Part A and/or Part B for Current Procedural Terminology [CPT] and Resource-Based Relative Value Scale [RBRVS]).

e. Processes to improve continuity of care, outcomes, and outcome measures.

Approved July 27, 2004, by the Academy of Managed Care Pharmacy, the American Association of Colleges of Pharmacy, the American College of Apothecaries, the American College of Clinical Pharmacy, the American Society of Consultant Pharmacists, the American Pharmacists Association, the American Society of Health-System Pharmacists, the National Association of Boards of Pharmacy,[b] the National Association of Chain Drug Stores, the National Community Pharmacists Association, and the National Council of State Pharmacy Association Executives.

a   In some situations, Medication Therapy Management services may be provided to the caregiver or other persons involved in the care of the patient.

b   Organization policy does not allow the National Association of Boards of Pharmacy to take a position on payment issues.

Source: Bluml BM. Definition of medication therapy management: development of professionwide consensus. J Am Pharm Assoc. 2005;45:566–72.

FIGURE 6-1

Patient Information Record for patients with asthma.

Sample Patient Information record

Date: _____ ❑ If checked, this form must be reviewed by the patient's physician before placing in patient file.

Patient: _____ Phone: H _____ W _____
         (last)   (first)   (mi)

Address: _____

Birthdate: _____ Age: _____ Member No. _____

Height: _____ inches Weight: _____ lb. Member Group No.: _____

Sex: F___ M ___ Pregnant: Y ___ N ___ Referring Physician _____

Physician provider No: _____

Past Medical History:

❑ Asthma	❑ Ear Infections	❑ Hay fever	❑ Liver disease	❑ Other _____
❑ Cancer	❑ Epilepsy	❑ Hypertension	❑ Thyroid disease	❑ Other _____
❑ Diabetes	❑ Glaucoma	❑ Kidney disease	❑ Ulcer	❑ Other _____

Drug Allergies:

Drug	When	Explanation	Drug	When	Explanation
❑ Penicillin	_____	_____	❑ Aspirin	_____	_____
❑ Sulfa	_____	_____	❑ Other	_____	_____

Prescription Medications Currently Taking:
(indicate if pm)

Drug	Strength	Sig	Compliance%	Last refill date	Drug	Strength	Sig	Compliance%	Last refill
___	___	___	___	___	___	___	___	___	___
___	___	___	___	___	___	___	___	___	___
___	___	___	___	___	___	___	___	___	___
___	___	___	___	___	___	___	___	___	___

OTC Medications Currently Taking: _____

Subjective: How is your asthma/breathing? _____ Correct use of:

How do you feel? _____ MDI   (Yes_No_N/A_)

Any new complaints? _____ Extender (Yes_No_N/A_)

Any problems with your medications? _____ Nebulizer (Yes_No_N/A_)

Notes: _____ PEFM (Yes_No_N/A_)

Objective: Serum levels of theophylline: Started

Level_____ meg/ml Date/time:_____ New Rx medications _____

Last drug, dose and time before level: _____ (since last visit) _____

Temp._____ Pulse_____ Resp._____ B/P_____ PEFR_____ New OTC medications _____

(since last visit) _____

Assessment: _____ Referred to Immediate Medical Care (_____)

_____

_____

_____

Plan: Goal/Desired Outcome/Basis of Recommendation: _____

Action Taken: _____

Recommendation(s): _____

_____

Follow-up:

Next scheduled visit (within 30 days; at refill time if possible)

Date: _____ Time: _____

Prepared by: (print) _____ Signature: _____ Phone: _____

Pharmacy: _____ Address: _____ NABP#: _____

Adapted from Pharmaceutical Care for Patients with Asthma: A Certificate Program for Pharmacists. Self-Study Learning Guide. Washington, DC: American Pharmaceutical Association; 2000.

same extent as more complicated patients. Recognizing the types of patients for whom pharmacists can make a great difference, pharmacists are focusing on five types of MTM programs within community pharmacy:

- Diabetes care
- Lipids care
- Asthma care
- Hypertension and cardiovascular care
- Immunizations

For the first four of these areas, monitoring involves measuring blood glucose levels, lipid profiles, respiratory function, and blood pressure.

FIGURE 6-2

Process of obtaining patient fingerstick for measuring blood components.

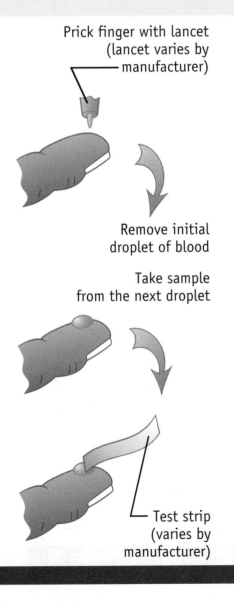

Prick finger with lancet (lancet varies by manufacturer)

Remove initial droplet of blood

Take sample from the next droplet

Test strip (varies by manufacturer)

BLOOD GLUCOSE LEVELS

The amount of glucose, or sugar, present in the blood (blood glucose levels) is generally measured directly from a blood sample obtained from a patient *fingerstick* (Figure 6-2). For the types of laboratory analyzers usually available in the pharmacy, *venipuncture* (drawing blood from a vein) is not needed. If you are helping to obtain the fingerstick or to analyze the blood for glucose, you must do so in accordance with the pharmacy's procedures and the analyzer's instructions. While dipsticks are still available in pharmacies for measuring glucose in patients' urine, this test is no longer viewed as clinically meaningful. The fingerstick, which with modern technology is relatively painless, helps pharmacists collect more useful information about blood glucose.

LIPID PROFILES

Simple analyzers available for measuring patients' *lipid levels* are also often available in pharmacies. Again, a fingerstick sample of blood is usually required for this analysis, although some analyzers require a venipuncture. Analyzers provide information about some or all of these lipid components of the blood: total cholesterol, triglycerides, low-density lipoproteins, and high-density lipoproteins. Ideally, the pharmacist needs all of these values to make an accurate assessment of patients' clinical condition. However, for the purpose of screening patients and referring those with high cholesterol to physicians, the pharmacist needs only total cholesterol.

RESPIRATORY FUNCTION

For patients with asthma, the most common means of measuring lung function outside a laboratory involves the peak flow meter (Figure 6-3). These devices are very convenient for patient use at home or for use in the pharmacy. They record peak expiratory flow (PEF), or the maximum amount of air the patient can blow out with one big breath. Measurements of PEF with peak flow meters are easy, practical, and inexpensive, making them perfect for short-term monitoring, managing exacerbations, and long-term monitoring by patients at home. Because reference values vary widely for different available meters, the patient must be taught to compare daily values with his or her "personal best" PEF value obtained with the same

FIGURE 6-3A

A Peak Flow Meter is the primary means of measuring lung function in patients with asthma outside hospital laboratories.

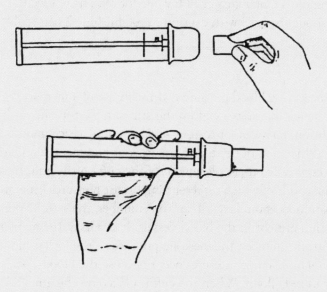

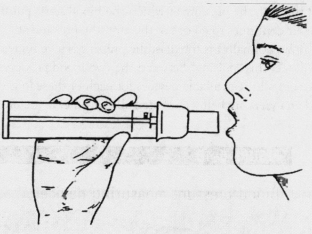

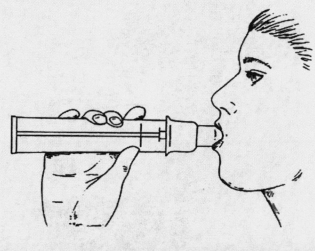

1. Make sure the peak flow arrow/indicator is at the bottom of the scale.

2. If there is a mouthpiece, attach it to the peak flow meter.

3. Hold the peak flow meter so that your fingers do not block the opening, indicator, or exhaust.

4. Breathe out and hold your breath for a few seconds.

5. Inhale as deeply as you can and place your mouth firmly around the mouthpiece, making sure your lips form a tight seal.

6. Blow out as hard and as fast as you can, in one big "gust".

7. Write down the number you get.

8. Repeat steps 1-7 two more times.

9. Choose the highest number of the three readings and compare with the predicted values or personal best.

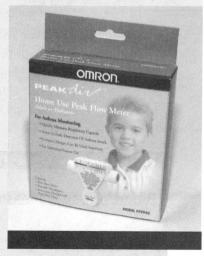

FIGURE 6-3B

Example of a commercially available Peak Flow Meter.

STORAGE AND MAINTENANCE:

Store the peak flow meter in the open air, not in a plastic bag. To clean, use a damp paper towel for the mouthpiece and the blowing tube, and dry completely. Do not put the whole meter under water! Please check the directions for your specific peak flow meter, including recommendations for replacing the device.

Source: Pharmaceutical Care for Patients with Asthma: A Certificate Program for Pharmacists. Self-Study Learning Guide. *Washington, DC: American Pharmaceutical Association; 2000.*

meter. Each patient's personal best PEF can most accurately be estimated during a 2- to 3-week period during which the patient records PEF two to four times per day. Once the patient's condition is stabilized, the personal best value is usually achieved in the early afternoon. Patients will occasionally observe a much greater PEF value for reasons not well understood. Such "outlier" values should be used with caution in establishing a personal best PEF.

BLOOD PRESSURE

The most accurate method of measuring blood pressure is through use of a mercury sphygmomanometer, which is the device that uses a cuff on the arm, a table-top unit with mercury, and a stethoscope. In addition, many easier-to-use—but not quite as accurate—devices are available (Figure 6-4). Whichever of these is in use in your pharmacy, familiarize yourself with its proper operation, especially proper placement of the cuff on the arm. Blood pressure is expressed as two numbers, both of which represent important pressures generated in the blood vessels as the heart contracts and relaxes. The "top" number, the systolic pressure, is the highest amount of pressure present in the blood vessels. It occurs at the moment when the heart contracts. The "bottom" number, the diastolic pressure, is the lowest blood pressure. It occurs when the heart relaxes. These pressures occur because the blood vessels are a closed system, just like water in a balloon. When the cuff is placed on the arm and pumped up, it stops the blood flowing in an artery just under the skin on the inside of the elbow. As the air is slowly let out of the cuff, the pressure at which the blood starts pulsing is the systolic pressure. Then, as the air continues to go out of the cuff, the pressure at which the blood stops pulsing (and flows normally) is the diastolic pressure. Have someone take your blood pressure, and you will feel this "pulsing" between the two blood pressures.

It is impossible to explain how to use all the available devices for each of these four measurements, and new devices and analyzers are being marketed all the time. If you are

FIGURE 6-4A

Blood pressure measuring device.

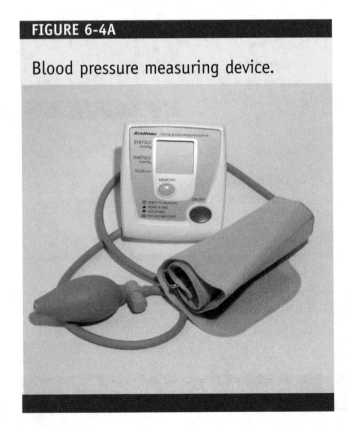

FIGURE 6-4B

Blood pressure measuring device.

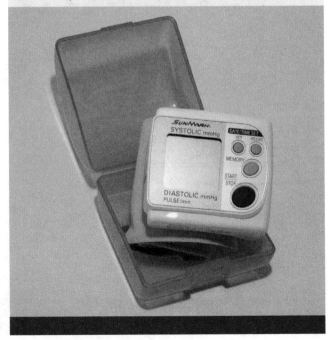

TABLE 6-3

Patient-Specific Information Needed for Medication Therapy Management and Pharmaceutical Care[a]

DEMOGRAPHIC INFORMATION

Name

Address

Telephone number, and perhaps e-mail address

Date of birth

Gender

Religion or religious affiliation

Occupation

ADMINISTRATIVE INFORMATION

Physicians and other prescribers

Pharmacy

Room/bed numbers (in hospitals, nursing homes, and other institutions)

Consent forms

Patient identification number

MEDICAL INFORMATION

Weight and height

Acute and chronic medical problems

Current symptoms

Vital signs and other monitoring information

Allergies and intolerances

Past medical history

Laboratory information

Diagnostic and surgical procedures

MEDICATION THERAPY REGIMEN

Prescription medications

Nonprescription medications

Medications used before, during, and after hospital/nursing facility stays

Home remedies, natural products, alternative medicines used

Adherence to therapy (how well the patient takes medications as directed; an older term is compliance)

Persistence with therapy (how well the patient comes back for needed refills of medications)

Medical allergies and intolerances

Concerns or questions about therapy

Assessment of understanding of therapy

Pertinent health beliefs

BEHAVIORAL AND LIFESTYLE INFORMATION

Diet

Exercise and recreation

Use of tobacco, alcohol, caffeine, and substances of abuse (illicit drugs)

Sexual history

Personality type

Daily activities

SOCIAL AND ECONOMIC INFORMATION

Living arrangement

Ethnic background

Financial, insurance, and health plan data

Originally published by the American Society of Health-System Pharmacists. ASHP guidelines on a standardized method for pharmaceutical care. *Am J Health Syst Pharm.* 1996;53:1713–1716. ©1996, American Society of Health-System Pharmacists, Inc. All rights reserved. Adapted with permission.

[a] Most of the information in this table is collected directly from the patient or a parent or other caregiver (in the case of children or people with dementia or other conditions that prevent them from being reliable sources of information). Some of the information is generated from pharmacy records (such as adherence and persistence), transferred from health records that may be obtained from other providers (such as a hospital or physician), or gathered by the pharmacist during physical assessment. Not all of the information is needed for every patient. But each of these categories of information can come into play in specific patients when certain diseases, conditions, or health situations are present.

Source: Bluml BM. Definition of medication therapy management: development of professionwide consensus. J Am Pharm Assoc. 2005;45:566–72.

involved in helping with these activities in your pharmacy, find out what devices are being used, and make sure that the pharmacist shows you exactly how to use them.

Assisting with Immunizations

As discussed above, the role of the pharmacist has expanded in many states to include injections. This has resulted in a proliferation of pharmacies offering immunizations, especially flu shots in the fall. Many pharmacists have been certified for immunizations, and

FIGURE 6-5

Durable medical equipment available in community pharmacies.

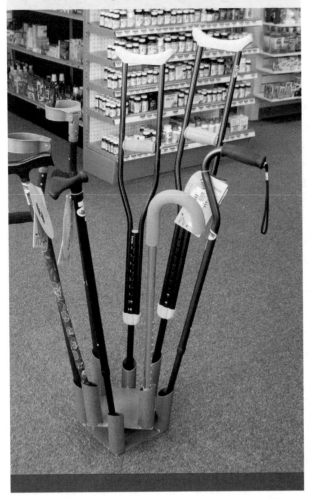

How patients respond to various medications (as well as nondrug therapies, such as improved diet or exercise) determines whether medication therapy should be continued, stopped, or altered.

they administer most of the flu shots in their pharmacies. In other states or situations, nurses work in the pharmacy during "flu shot days" or at specified times to give flu shots and other immunizations.

During these times, you as a pharmacy technician may be called on to assist with registering patients, ensuring that the necessary information about the patient and his or her medical history is available, and making sure patients remain in the pharmacy after their shot long enough to detect any adverse reactions. Discuss your role with the pharmacist so that you are certain you know what is expected of you and how to perform the tasks you are asked to help with.

Assisting with Medical Appliances and Devices

Many pharmacists have built extensive businesses in the field of durable medical equipment or DME. Ostomy products, canes, crutches, and home infusion and respiratory equipment are among the wide variety of goods that fall into this category (Figures 6-5 and 6-6).

DME is attractive from a business standpoint because its cost is often reimbursable to the pharmacy under the federal government's Medicare Part A program (see Chapters 3 and 11). The Medicare program covers elderly and disabled Americans. When patients need the kinds of products listed above, Medicare Part A pays health care providers, including pharmacies, to provide them.

For you as a pharmacy technician, DME may be an important part of your job. However, because of its specialized nature, pharmacists usually handle most of the activities themselves. These functions include:

- Measuring patients to fit them with devices such as ostomy products; canes, crutches, and walkers; and wheelchairs. Patients who need ostomy products have usually had cancer and as a result require alternative portals for excrement. The most common situation is colon cancer that requires surgical removal of the last part of the colon, including the anus. In this case, the remaining colon is rerouted to a position on the patient's side, where an ostomy bag can be attached to collect wastes.
- Educating patients about the device they are using. Home infusion equipment is used by patients to self-administer fluids, medications, or both on a long-term basis. These infusions are generally running into the patient's veins (intravenous infusions), but some patients also receive peritoneal dialysis at home. In this case, large volumes of fluids are infused into the peritoneal cavity (the space around the patient's large organs [stomach, liver, intestines]). The fluid can draw out many of the wastes from the blood flowing through these organs, hence the term dialysis.
- Making sterile products for home administration to patients. This is a key area where many pharmacy technicians are involved in DME. The process by which you will make intravenous infusions, peritoneal dialysis fluids, and total parenteral nutrition (TPN) products is explained in Chapter 10. TPN is a specialized type of infusion that contains nutrients for patients who are unable to eat foods or drink liquids. TPN, which is still occasionally referred to by its older name of

hyperalimentation, contains high concentrations of sugars and amino acids along with vitamins, minerals, and trace elements. TPN solutions are often administered to patients continuously, and they are given through a special administration port placed into a large vein just before it reaches the heart (this is called a central line to differentiate it from normal intravenous sites, which are called peripheral lines). Fat emulsions are given with TPN several times each week to help the patient get the oils and fats needed in a healthy diet.

Conclusion

By assisting the pharmacist with both dispensing and pharmaceutical care activities, you can become a valuable and necessary part of the pharmacy. The primary tool you will use to complete these tasks is the computer. Let's look at Chapter 7 to learn how pharmacy has adapted to life in the Information Age of the 21st century.

For More Information

If you are preparing for the Pharmacy Technician Certification Examination and feel that you need more information about the topics discussed in this chapter, consider studying these sources of additional information:

- Medication Therapy Management Services in the Community Pharmacy: Planning for Successful Implementation, published by APhA.
- The references listed for this chapter.
- Snipe K. Pharmacy technician job description and duties. In: *The Pharmacy Technician Skills-Building Manual*. Washington, D.C.: American Pharmacists Association; 2007: 1-8.
- American Pharmacists Association. *Pharmacist Disease Management: Diabetes*. 3rd ed. Washington, D.C.: American Pharmacists Association; 2005.
- Rovers JP, Currie JD. *A Practical Guide to Pharmaceutical Care*. 3rd ed. Washington, D.C.: American Pharmacists Association; 2007.

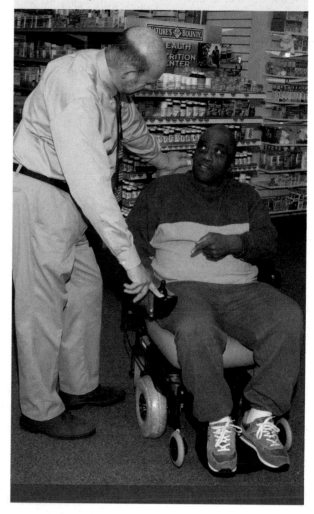

FIGURE 6-6

Pharmacist counseling a patient about wheelchairs in a community pharmacy.

The role of the pharmacist has expanded in many states to include injections.

References

American Society of Health-System Pharmacists. ASHP guidelines on a standardized method for pharmaceutical care. *Am J Health Syst Pharm.* 1996;53:1713–6.

Angaran DM. Quality assurance to quality improvement: measuring and monitoring pharmaceutical care. *Am J Hosp Pharm.* 1991;48:1901–7.

Bluml BM, McKenney JM, Cziraky MJ. Pharmaceutical care services and results in Project ImPACT: hyperlipidemia. *J Am Pharm Assoc.* 2000;40:157–65.

Bootman JL. The $76 billion wake-up call. *J Am Pharm Assoc.* 1996;NS36:27–8.

Cranor CW, Bunting BA, Christensen DB. Long-term clinical and economic outcomes in a community pharmacy diabetes care program: the Asheville project. *J Am Pharm Assoc.* 2003;43:173–84.

Cranor CW, Christensen DB. Factors associated with outcomes among patients with diabetes enrolled in an employer-sponsored pharmaceutical care service: the Asheville project. *J Am Pharm Assoc.* 2003;43:160–72.

Cranor CW, Christensen DB. Short-term outcomes of a community pharmacy diabetes care program: the Asheville project. *J Am Pharm Assoc.* 2003;43:149–59.

Day RL, Goyan JE, Herfindal ET, et al. The origins of the clinical pharmacy program at the University of California, San Francisco. *DICP Ann Pharmacother.* 1991;25:308–14.

Ernst FR, Grizzle AJ. Drug-related morbidity and mortality: updating the cost-of-illness model. *J Am Pharm Assoc.* 2001:41:192–8.

Garrett DG, Martin LA. The Asheville project: participants' perceptions of factors contributing to the success of a patient self-management diabetes program. *J Am Pharm Assoc.* 2003;43:185–90.

Hepler CD. Pharmacy as a clinical profession. *Am J Hosp Pharm.* 1985; 42:1298–306.

Hepler CD. The third wave in pharmaceutical education: The clinical movement. *Am J Pharm Educ.* 1987;51:369–85.

Hepler CD, Strand LM. Opportunities and responsibilities in pharmaceutical care. *Am J Pharm Educ.* 1989;53(suppl):7S–15S.

Hepler CD, Strand LM. Opportunities and responsibilities in pharmaceutical care. *Am J Pharm Educ.* 1990; 47:543–9.

Hogue MD, Grabenstein JD, Foster SL, Rothholz MC. Pharmacist involvement with immunizations: a decade of professional achievement. *J Am Pharm Assoc.* 2006;46:168–82.

Johnson JA, Bootman JL. Drug-related morbidity and mortality: a cost-of-illness model. *Arch Intern Med* 1995;155:1949–56.

Penna RP. Pharmaceutical care: Pharmacy's mission for the 1990s. *Am J Hosp Pharm.* 1990;47:543–9.

Study Commission on Pharmacy. *Pharmacists for the Future.* Ann Arbor, MI: Health Administration Press; 1975:139–43.

CHAPTER SEVEN

Pharmacy Computer Systems and Automation

With the rapid pace of progress in the field of pharmacy computers and automated dispensing systems, it is not possible to present timely information on specific products and systems in a textbook. Rather, this chapter describes the importance of such systems in contemporary pharmacy practice and describes some of the practical problems their introduction has caused, including the challenges automation and computers present to regulatory authorities.

FIGURE 7-1

Hospital pharmacist using a computer for a variety of tasks.

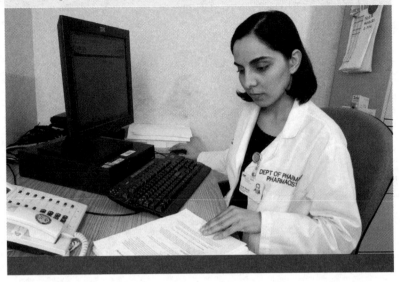

Pharmacy is probably the most computerized part of the health care world.

Introduction

Pharmacy is probably the most computerized part of the health care world. Everything from patients' prescriptions to drug inventories to patient-education materials are maintained on computer (Figure 7-1). In most hospitals and many busier community pharmacies, automated dispensing machines and robotic devices assist in drug-dispensing activities day in and day out.

But, as people have discovered with personal computers, these wonderful devices have not reduced the number of hours people work each week. If anything, computers and our electronic global village—with its Web and e-mail messages—have made the workweek a 24/7 proposition. Likewise, computers and computer technology will create jobs and opportunities for you as a pharmacy technician, provided you learn how to use them.

The purpose of this chapter is to describe the basic types of computerized systems that are available for dispensing and patient care activities. In addition, you will need to learn the specifics of the computer technology used in your practice setting either on the job or in special training classes.

Computerized Systems for Pharmacy Dispensing

Pharmacists have been using computer technology for prescription processing and dispensing since the late 1970s. Prescription records are perfect for database storage, because a few discrete fields completely describe each transaction. These fields are listed in Table 7-1.

By having computerized order entry as the first step in prescription dispensing, pharmacists have been able to use the computer to assist in such important tasks as checking for drug interactions with other drugs, foods, diseases, or laboratory tests; evaluating patient conditions that would preclude use of the prescribed drug; and detailing special precautions needed when this patient is using this particular drug. Because the computer cannot yet judge the relevance of this information to a certain patient, the pharmacist must apply his or her own knowledge to decide what action to take when the computer "flags" a prescription as having a potential problem.

Computerized order entry screens (Figure 7-2) use codes for drug names and strengths as well as instructions for use. While it may take time to become accustomed to these codes, they greatly speed the rate at which you can

FIGURE 7-2

Pharmacy Computer Order Entry Screen.

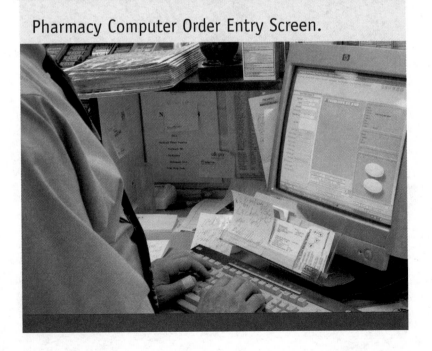

enter prescriptions into the system without having to type out everything in full. These prescription systems have been around almost as long as personal computers, but automated and robotic equipment has created much excitement among pharmacists. The types of computer-related technology now in routine use include the following:

- **Automated prescription-dispensing systems —**
  For community pharmacies, *automated prescription-dispensing systems* (Figure 7-3) fill one half or more of the daily workload in the pharmacy department. The process begins when orders are entered into prescription software systems by the technician and the actual prescription scanned into the system. Using drug products that are placed into bins—usually by technicians—these robotic-like devices interpret the prescription order, prepare a label, place medication into a vial or other container, and transfer the prescription label onto the container. The pharmacist then checks the entire process and uses computer-generated patient-counseling materials to make sure the patient knows how to take the medication properly.

- **Automated cart-fill machines —**
  A similar type of machine used in hospital and nursing home operations is the *automated cart-fill machine*. In institutions, medications are often transferred from the pharmacy to the patient-care areas using carts. These carts have drawers, called cassettes. Each cassette contains the medications ordered by the physician for one patient for a given period of time (usually 24 hours in a hospital, but up to 30 days for a long-term care facility such as a nursing home). The automated cart-fill machine picks the drugs that are on each patient's computerized profile from medication bins filled by pharmacy technicians. It then places the correct number of medications into the patient's cassette. These automated systems rely on bar codes to be certain that the right medication is being prepared based on each prescription order.

- **Automated point-of-care dispensing machines —**
  Another type of technology in use in institutions is the *automated point-of-care dispensing machine*, often called the Pyxis, after the company that markets it. The machines are placed in patient-care areas where nurses can obtain some of the medications needed for each patient directly from the machine. A common use for these point-of-care devices is to store controlled substances, those medications that can be abused (see Chapter 3). Because these types of drugs cannot be placed in the unlocked cassettes on the carts (from which they could be easily "diverted" for personal use

---

TABLE 7-1

Prescription Records in a Database

A prescription record in a database includes the following fields:

- Date
- Patient name and address (often stored in a separate patient database)
- Drug name and dosage (often stored in a separate drug database)
- Quantity
- Directions for use
- Refills
- Prescriber name and address (also often stored in a separate prescriber database)
- Patient education and counseling information (stored in the drug or a related database)
- Patient prescription history (stored in the prescription database or some other related database)

FIGURE 7-3

Robotic Prescription Dispensing System.

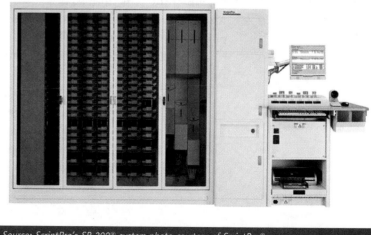

Source: ScriptPro's SP 200® system photo courtesy of ScriptPro®.

As computerized
technology becomes
more sophisticated, it
will be used to
perform tasks that
humans now do.

Computers and our
electronic global
village—with its
Web and e-mail
messages—have
made the workweek
a 24/7 proposition.

Two needs of MTM
services match
perfectly with the
capabilities of
computer programs:
documentation
and billing.

or for illegal sale "on the street"), the point-of-care machines restrict access to the medications and require the nurse to record the name of the patient who is to receive each dose.

- **Robots for product delivery —**
  Finally, automated devices are used, primarily in very large hospitals, for delivering medications to patient-care areas. These machines are robots, just like you might see in movies. They roll through the halls, getting on and off elevators, and talk to people that they sense nearby. On the nursing unit, they "deliver" patient medications to nurses, recording who accepted transfer of the drugs. The robots can be very useful in hospitals that do not have other less expensive delivery mechanisms, such as pneumatic tube systems. Just like drive-in banking centers, pneumatic tubes are used in many hospitals to bring medication orders to the pharmacy and to send medications to the patient-care areas.

As automated systems develop in the 21st century, they will surely present more challenges and opportunities to pharmacists and technicians. As computerized technology becomes more sophisticated, it will be used to perform tasks that humans now do. Increasingly, the job of humans will be to program, manage, fill, and repair automated systems. As a pharmacy technician, you may find yourself becoming more of a computer technician in the years ahead.

Computerized Systems for Medication Therapy Management Activities

Just as information technology is an essential feature of pharmacy-dispensing processes, computers are increasingly important in medication therapy management (MTM) services as well. In several key areas, pharmacists are using technology to manage clinical tasks and information. Two needs of MTM services match perfectly with the capabilities of computer programs: documentation and billing. Documentation is the recording of information about the patient and the interventions made by the pharmacist and other pharmacy personnel. This record keeping is essential for two reasons. First, to be paid by third-party payers, the pharmacist must have a record of the work performed. Second, if something goes wrong and the patient later becomes ill or dies, the pharmacist will need to have information that can be presented in court to show that the interventions made were necessary and appropriate.

Billing, which is covered in more detail in Chapter 11, is the process of obtaining payment from insurance companies, the government, or health plans. Pharmacy owners sign contracts with these third-party payers, and the contract requires the pharmacy to keep records of the prescriptions dispensed and other interventions made. The records must be made available to the third-party payer on demand so that the payer can be sure that the pharmacy has in fact done what it has been paid for. These records are critically important to avoid contract cancellation or criminal charges that the pharmacy has defrauded the third-party payer.

For pharmaceutical care, many types of information are recorded in computer software programs. This information is listed in Table 7-2.

If you are asked to enter pharmaceutical care information into the computer, you will need to complete training for the systems used in your workplace.

Computer-Related Issues in Pharmacy Practice

Information today is a very powerful—and valuable—commodity. But just as people are concerned about companies sharing or selling information about their credit card transactions, they are troubled to learn that their pharmacy provides information to outside parties. This practice has become a part of a broader discussion of confidentiality with respect to health care information. Confidentiality is discussed in more detail in Chapter 8 but a brief mention is merited here with respect to computers.

The data available in pharmacy computer systems is of interest to several outside parties, but its confidentiality must be respected. If patients cannot share private information with their pharmacists without fear that other people or outside companies will learn about it, then they are not likely to tell the pharmacist everything necessary for pharmacists to provide quality pharmaceutical care. Pharmacies have sometimes encountered public outcry or lawsuits when they have engaged in the following practices:

- Using pharmaceutical industry grants to pay outside companies to send prescription refill reminders to patients
- Providing names and addresses of patients who have had prescriptions filled for certain drugs to the manufacturers of those or competing drugs, and providing the names of prescribing physicians to manufacturers

---

TABLE 7-2

Pharmaceutical Care Information in Computer Software Programs

Types of pharmaceutical care information recorded in computer software programs include:

- **Care plans** (what problems the pharmacist has found and how they are to be treated)
- **Disease management** (interventions unique to various diseases)
- **Therapeutic outcomes** (the effects of interventions on the patient's clinical condition as well as quality of life)
- **Progress notes** (what the pharmacist observes in each visit with the patient)
- **Billing information** (when and how payment was requested)

Conclusion

While the cold, impersonal computer may have become the workhorse of the pharmacy, you must never forget the "people" side of pharmacy practice. Everything you do is aimed at producing positive effects on people's lives. In your role as a pharmacy technician, you will interact with patients—who are in all respects the reason the pharmacy was established and continues to operate—and with the health professionals who take care of these patients. In Chapter 8, let's look at ways of communicating with and pleasing the important people you deal with every day.

For More Information

If you are preparing for the Pharmacy Technician Certification Examination and feel that you need more information about the topics discussed in this chapter, consider studying these sources of additional information:

- ComputerTalk for the Pharmacist
  http://www.amazon.com/Computer-Talk-for-the-Pharmacist/dp/B00006K9TY
- Snipe K. Automated systems. In: *The Pharmacy Technician Skills-Building Manual.* Washington, D.C.: American Pharmacists Association; 2007:143–8.

If patients cannot share private information with their pharmacists without fear that other people or outside companies will learn about it, then they are not likely to tell the pharmacist everything necessary for pharmacists to provide quality pharmaceutical care.

CHAPTER EIGHT

Interacting
with Patients

Appropriate communications with patients is the theme of Chapter 8, which introduces legally mandated counseling by pharmacists and defines the role of the technician. This chapter briefly describes techniques for handling patients with special communication requirements, including those with terminal illnesses and those who become belligerent. The chapter discusses confidentiality of patient information, summarizes a court case that involved a pharmacy technician, and discusses provisions of a federal law that protects the confidentiality of patients' health information.

Introduction

Regardless of the role you play and the type of pharmacy you work in, you will be called on to interact with other people. In a community pharmacy, most communications will likely be with patients and the people you work with. In a hospital or long-term care facility, you may most commonly communicate with health care professionals such as physicians and nurses. But no matter where you work and what you're doing, these communications with other people will be a major determinant of how you are viewed as you do your job.

This chapter details communications with patients. However, think broadly as you read this material because much of it applies to communications with any of the people you encounter during your daily activities as a pharmacy technician. Without positive communications with other people, your prescription-filling efforts and your contribution to the overall operation of the pharmacy will likely be overlooked. Unless people sense a warm, caring, and empathic attitude, they may overlook how well you are performing or how much you know. As a speaker told a chain-pharmacy audience, "I don't care how much you know until I know how much you care."

Understanding the Definitions and Principles of Communication

In its simplest form, communication is the process of conveying information from one person to another. In the case of spoken communication, one person says something (a process called encoding), and someone hears and interprets it (decoding). If the communication has been effective, the second person will have received the same message that the first person sent. The second person may then respond, and the first person uses this information (feedback) to assess whether the correct message was received.

In this process, there is much room for error. You probably have seen what happens to a message when it is passed around the members of a group—it becomes distorted as people place their own interpretations on what was said and then pass it along "in their own

---

TABLE 8-1

Principles of Communication

Four major principles associated with the process of communication are:

- **Communication can be intentional or unintentional.** When talking with patients, you must be careful not to convey unintentional messages of indifference, anger, or frustration—and these messages can come from the way you stand, look, or behave during the interaction.

- **It is impossible not to communicate.** Even when you stand and listen to someone else, not saying anything, the speaker is reading your face, your hands, and your body for nonverbal clues of agreement or understanding or emotions such as anger or happiness. When dealing with patients, pharmacists and technicians must communicate an air of trustworthiness and concern so that effective communications can occur.

- **Communication is irreversible.** Once something has been said, it can never be erased. Like an arrow from a bow, you cannot pull back the words once you have released them. You can apologize, but the damage will remain the same. When talking with patients, there is no room for error, unprofessional attitudes, or indifference.

- **Communication is unrepeatable.** Every encounter is completely new. What worked on one patient may not work on the next. What worked this month may not work when the same patient is counseled next month. Effective communication in health care depends not on a set of standardized words and phrases but on a set of general guidelines for communication. These guidelines reflect an appreciation for the process of encoding, decoding, and feedback and an understanding of these principles of communication.

words." Based on the feedback the sender of a message receives, the sender may restate the message in other words and ask the recipient to repeat what he or she has heard. This process of encoding, decoding, and feedback can continue until both parties feel they have the same message.

In addition, people interpret nonverbal clues—such as facial expressions, hand motions, and the way the body is positioned—as they are decoding messages. For instance, if someone gives off nonverbal clues of being dishonest, the recipient of the message may not believe the person. Or if a person laughs while conveying serious information, the recipient may be confused about what the real message is. Suppose someone just diagnosed with diabetes yawned during a 30-minute patient-education session about the disease—you would wonder why he is bored when he should be receiving valuable information that could affect his future health.

People also glean a lot of information from the written word and from pictures or graphics that accompany those words. To increase the chance that patients will understand what their medications are used for and how the medications are to be used, pharmacists routinely provide patients with informative flyers that explain the medication in both words and diagrams. While the above description of communication is useful from a learning standpoint, the linear process described often seems rare in the real world. Instead, both parties may be trying to communicate with each other while ignoring each other's messages as they struggle to get their own messages across. So what is communication? Here is one brief definition: Communication is the process of interaction between participants who occupy different but overlapping environments and create a relationship by exchanging messages, many of which may be blocked by "noise."

Principles associated with the process of communication are discussed in Table 8-1.

Communicating with Patients

In an encounter with a patient, you must first be aware of the purpose of the interaction. Are you trying to gather information from the patient (name, address, allergies to medications), or are you trying to convey information to the patient (when the prescription will be ready, whether the patient wants to be counseled by the pharmacist)?

When you are trying to gather information from patients, different types of questions are effective in different types of situations (Table 8-2).

When seeking information from a patient, you must listen carefully. Be aware of whether the patient is answering the questions completely and accurately. If the patient appears to be changing the subject or trying to get across information other than what you are asking for, listen to what he or she is saying. Perhaps the patient has an existing relationship with the pharmacist or someone else in the pharmacy; if so, call on that person to help. If the patient is describing some problem other than the one you are asking about, listen to the message, repeat it back to the patient, and then take an appropriate action.

TABLE 8-2

Questions to Help You Gather Information

Some types of questions that may be effective for information-gathering include:

- **Open-ended questions**—those that cannot be answered with a "yes" or "no" ("Since you began this medicine for high blood pressure last month, how have you been feeling?")

- **Closed-ended questions**—those that can be answered with a "yes" or "no" ("Did you finish all your medication last month?")

- **Direct questions**—those that ask for the desired information in a straightforward manner ("Do you feel better or worse when you're taking this medication?")

- **Indirect questions**—questions or even statements that disguise the actual information being sought by calling for a general response from the other party ("I'm wondering how you've been doing on this new medication.")

FIGURE 8-1

The OTC "Drug Facts" Label.

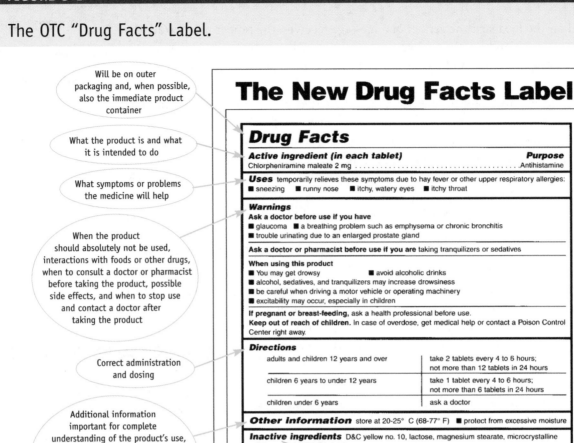

Will be on outer packaging and, when possible, also the immediate product container

What the product is and what it is intended to do

What symptoms or problems the medicine will help

When the product should absolutely not be used, interactions with foods or other drugs, when to consult a doctor or pharmacist before taking the product, possible side effects, and when to stop use and contact a doctor after taking the product

Correct administration and dosing

Additional information important for complete understanding of the product's use, including information for consumers who may be allergic to certain ingredients (e.g., aspartame) or who must restrict the intake of dietary ingredients (e.g., sodium)

Standard placement will help consumers who must watch inactive ingredients

The New Drug Facts Label

Drug Facts

Active ingredient (in each tablet) **Purpose**
Chlorpheniramine maleate 2 mg . . . . .Antihistamine

Uses temporarily relieves these symptoms due to hay fever or other upper respiratory allergies:
■ sneezing ■ runny nose ■ itchy, watery eyes ■ itchy throat

Warnings
Ask a doctor before use if you have
■ glaucoma ■ a breathing problem such as emphysema or chronic bronchitis
■ trouble urinating due to an enlarged prostate gland

Ask a doctor or pharmacist before use if you are taking tranquilizers or sedatives

When using this product
■ You may get drowsy ■ avoid alcoholic drinks
■ alcohol, sedatives, and tranquilizers may increase drowsiness
■ be careful when driving a motor vehicle or operating machinery
■ excitability may occur, especially in children

If pregnant or breast-feeding, ask a health professional before use.
Keep out of reach of children. In case of overdose, get medical help or contact a Poison Control Center right away.

Directions

adults and children 12 years and over	take 2 tablets every 4 to 6 hours; not more than 12 tablets in 24 hours
children 6 years to under 12 years	take 1 tablet every 4 to 6 hours; not more than 6 tablets in 24 hours
children under 6 years	ask a doctor

Other information store at 20-25° C (68-77° F) ■ protect from excessive moisture

Inactive ingredients D&C yellow no. 10, lactose, magnesium stearate, microcrystalline cellulose, pregelatinized starch

---

TABLE 8-3

Checking Patients' Understanding

You should make sure the patient can repeat back to you information you have presented, including:

• Name of the drug

• What it is being used for

• How often the medication is taken

• How the medication is used (apply, insert, swallow, inject)

• What to do if a dose is missed

Suppose you are working in the prescription department and a young woman brings a bottle of liquid cough and cold medication to you. She asks if this product is good for fever, in addition to coughs and head congestion. At this point, you need information, perhaps from both the patient and the pharmacist. First you need to gather information by asking the patient several questions, including who will use the product (her, her husband, her children, a friend) and what symptoms the ill person has (Is the nose runny or stopped up? How high is the fever? Is the cough productive? How long have these symptoms been present?) This information-gathering step is very critical to your ability to answer the woman's question. Without it, your response could be inappropriate, incorrect, or just plain meaningless.

When you are giving information to a patient, ask him or her to repeat the information back to you. For instance, when counseling a patient, the pharmacist should make sure the patient can restate information such as that in Table 8-3.

FIGURE 8-2

An Example of a Dietary Supplement Label as Required
by the Food and Drug Administration.

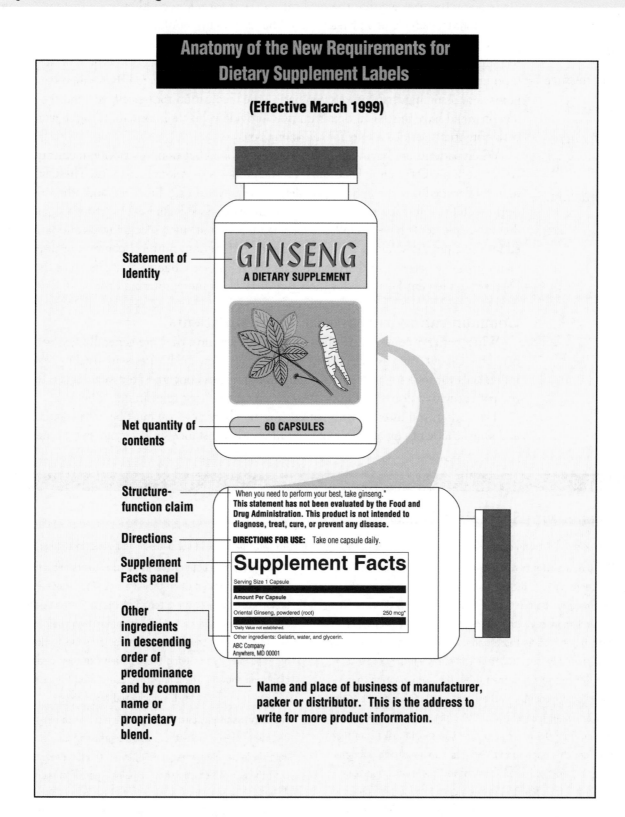

Anatomy of the New Requirements for Dietary Supplement Labels

(Effective March 1999)

GINSENG
A DIETARY SUPPLEMENT

Statement of Identity

Net quantity of contents — 60 CAPSULES

Structure-function claim — When you need to perform your best, take ginseng.* **This statement has not been evaluated by the Food and Drug Administration. This product is not intended to diagnose, treat, cure, or prevent any disease.**

Directions — **DIRECTIONS FOR USE:** Take one capsule daily.

Supplement Facts panel

Supplement Facts

Serving Size 1 Capsule

Amount Per Capsule

Oriental Ginseng, powdered (root)	250 mcg*

*Daily Value not established.

Other ingredients: Gelatin, water, and glycerin.

ABC Company
Anywhere, MD 00001

Other ingredients in descending order of predominance and by common name or proprietary blend.

Name and place of business of manufacturer, packer or distributor. This is the address to write for more product information.

If the patient is describing some problem other than the one you are asking about, listen to the message, repeat it back to the patient, and then take an appropriate action.

In the above example of the young woman with the cough-and-cold remedy, suppose she tells you that the medication is for a 3-year-old boy who has had a fever of 103°F for 4 days. You read on the package that the medication is not for use in children younger than 6 years old without the advice of a physician and that it does not contain any drug that would reduce fever. You should at this point consult with the pharmacist, who would likely recommend that the woman take the child to the doctor immediately because of the high fever and his young age. In this example, if you had merely answered the woman's question, perhaps by assuming that she was purchasing the medication for herself, you and the pharmacist would have missed an opportunity to provide valuable information to the woman—with potentially serious results for the young boy.

When patients are buying or seeking information about nonprescription medications, you can use the OTC Drug Facts label on the products to guide discussions. These labels list in a standardized way the active ingredient(s), uses, warnings, direction, and other information needed to safely use nonprescription medications (see Figure 8-1). Products approved as dietary supplements have a similar label (Figure 8-2), but since specific uses cannot be stated for these products, labels will contain structure-function, nutrient-content, or disease claims to guide patients in their purchasing decisions (see Chapter 3 discussion of the Dietary Supplement Health Education Act of 1994 for more information).

Communicating with Special Types of Patients

When patients come to the pharmacy for medications, they are generally sick or concerned about some aspect of their health. Only a few medications are used in healthy individuals without any immediate or overriding health concerns. In psychological terms, the patient with a disease is said to have taken on the "sick role" in our society.

Thus, when you interact with patients in the pharmacy, you must be both cognizant of and sympathetic or empathic about their illness. For instance, it is very inappropriate to

---

TABLE 8-4

Patients with Specialized Concerns

Pharmacists and technicians must be aware of the ways they communicate with patients in specialized situations, including:

- **The dying patient:** While most people who are facing death say there really is little that others can say to help them, they greatly appreciate the chance to say how they are feeling and know that others care enough to listen. Dying patients, especially those who have been long-term clients of a pharmacy, should not be ignored when they come to this difficult phase in their lives. The main emotion that you should recognize in these patients is fear—fear of pain, fear of dying, fear of death. Dying patients also need information from the pharmacist, and you should make sure that they get this opportunity. Patients who are taking pain and other medications need to know how the medications can be used safely, how to manage side effects such as drowsiness and vomiting, and whether they can continue activities such as driving a car.

- **The angry or uncooperative patient:** Patients become angry and frustrated when they are sick. They may be facing lifelong disability or life-altering diseases. These patients are often consumed by the loss of control over their lives and the fear that they will be dependent on medication or other people. By involving these patients in their treatment plans and showing them how they can control the disease, you can help dissipate this anger and frustration.

- **The depressed patient:** Some people respond to news of disease by becoming withdrawn or depressed. You can best help these people by frequently having short conversations with them in which you show genuine interest in their condition and express hope that they will get better. Such interactions help depressed patients overcome their feelings of helplessness.

close a purchase with a patient in a pharmacy by saying, "Come back again soon." This comment, while common in other retail stores, has a totally different meaning in a pharmacy: "We're glad you're sick. We hope you keep suffering so that we can make more money off your misfortune."

Because of their illness, patients may be facing their own impending death or the passing of a loved one, life-changing sickness that will require them to take medications for the rest of their lives, or anger about "why did this happen to me?" You need to be able to recognize certain patient types and develop communication strategies that will enable you to communicate with these people despite their other concerns, as discussed in Table 8-4.

Distributing Medications and Providing Patient Counseling and Education

If part of your job is to hand the completed prescription to the patient (and/or collect the money for the prescription), then you must be aware of several important issues. These include storage of the medication before distribution, information you can provide to the patient, and legal requirements about information the pharmacist must provide to the patient. In the retail setting, handling money will also be important.

Medication Storage

The storage of medications, a very important issue, is the subject of much attention in the pharmacy world (see Chapter 13). An increasing number of medications must be stored at specific temperatures (such as frozen, refrigerated, or room temperature). The medications are generally stored at the specified temperature all the way through the drug-distribution system—from manufacturer to wholesaler to pharmacy to patient. However, some medications that are refrigerated in the pharmacy may be stored at room temperature by the patient if they are to be taken over only a few days (such as an antibiotic).

Because of storage considerations, you should ensure the following:

- Once a prescription is prepared, it should be stored at the proper temperature in the pharmacy until it is delivered to the patient. For instance, if a prescription or refill is called in, but the patient does not pick up the medication for a few hours or days, it should be stored properly until the patient arrives.
- When you hand prescriptions to patients, be sure they understand how to store medications when they get home. Be certain patients understand the difference between frozen ("keep this in your freezer, where your ice is") and refrigerated ("keep this in your refrigerator, where you put your milk").
- If a prescription is being delivered by car, mail, or other carrier, it must not be exposed to extreme temperatures (such as left in a hot car during the summer) or kept outside its normal storage temperature for more than 24 hours. You may need to pack refrigerated or frozen drugs in an insulated container—perhaps even one containing ice or dry ice (Figure 8-3)—if delicate drug products are being shipped.

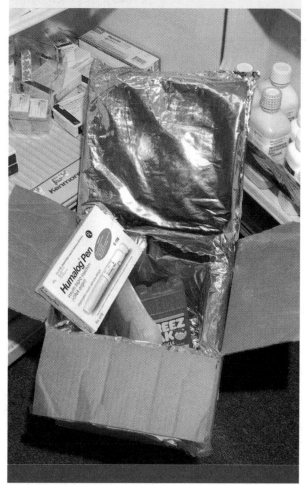

FIGURE 8-3

Packing a shipment box for medications that must remain under refrigeration (2–8°C).

The storage of medications, a very important issue, is the subject of much attention in the pharmacy world.

Information for the Patient

When you are giving prescriptions to patients, you are required under most state laws and the Omnibus Budget Reconciliation Act of 1990 (OBRA '90) to ask whether the person wants the pharmacist to counsel them about their prescription. In some chain pharmacies, the patient even signs a log book when they pick up the prescription, indicating whether or not they are requesting counseling. When patients sign such a book, make sure they understand what they are signing, as many patients think they are simply acknowledging receipt of their medications and do not realize they are giving up their legally mandated opportunity to receive counseling by the pharmacist.

As discussed in Chapter 3, OBRA '90 requires the pharmacist to offer to discuss with the patient or caregiver the following information:

- Name and description of the medication
- Dosage form, dose, route of administration, and duration of drug therapy
- Special directions and precautions for preparation, administration, and use of the medication by the patient
- Common or severe side effects, adverse reactions or interactions, and therapeutic contraindications that may be encountered, including ways of avoiding them, and the action required if they occur
- Techniques for self-monitoring of drug therapy
- Proper storage
- Prescription refill information
- Action to be taken in the event of a missed dose

In addition, the pharmacist is required under OBRA '90 to record and maintain the following information:

- Patient's name, address, telephone number, date of birth (or age), and sex
- Patient's individual history when important, including diseases, known allergies and drug reactions, and a comprehensive list of medications and relevant medical devices
- Pharmacist's comments about the individual's drug therapy

If patients state that they do not want counseling but then proceed to ask you questions about the prescription, be very cautious in your responses.

If patients state that they do not want counseling but then proceed to ask you questions about the prescription, be very cautious in your responses. While you can easily provide straightforward information such as the name of the drug, how it is taken and stored, and whether it can be refilled, ask the pharmacist to respond to queries involving what the drug is for, what side effects or adverse reactions may occur, and what to do if a dose is missed. While you certainly will learn many of these things in your work as a pharmacy technician, these questions are best handled by the pharmacist for legal, ethical, and practical reasons.

Cash Handling in the Retail Setting

If your job entails handling money in the pharmacy, you must take precautions to be sure this does not cause any problems. As in all retail settings, pharmacy owners and managers take seriously any discrepancies or perceived problems regarding the proper handling of money in their stores.

While it is beyond the scope of this text to provide detailed information on cash handling, keep in mind the tips discussed in Table 8-5.

Ensuring Confidentiality

Working in health care gives you access to some of the deepest secrets of people's lives: whether they are sexually active, whether they have an embarrassing disease, whether they have acquired immunodeficiency syndrome (AIDS). You must keep such information confidential and use it only in the course of your job as a pharmacy technician. Otherwise, you could not only hurt your patients and their loved ones but also find yourself and your employer in court facing civil lawsuits. In addition, pharmacies face penalties under the Health Insurance Portability and Accountability Act (HIPAA).

Simply put, there is no acceptable reason to discuss outside your job anything that you learn while working as a pharmacy technician about people and the medications they are taking. Even in situations where you may believe that a person has a disease such as AIDS and has not informed his or her spouse, your legal duty to the patient precludes you from telling the spouse, even if the spouse is also a patient in the pharmacy.

One court case involved a pharmacy technician who told her son that a patient had AIDS. While at school, the son teased the patient's child about the disease. The patient had never told the child about this fatal condition and sued both the pharmacy and the technician for damages. The case was settled out of court for an undisclosed amount.

HIPAA defines under federal law what constitutes "protected health information," or PHI, including documents kept on paper or in electronic form and oral communications. Health providers, including most pharmacies, must give patients a written "Notice of Privacy Practice," and they must not disclose PHI unless treatment, payment, or health care operations are involved or they have patient permission to disclose information outside these areas. Pharmacies and other health providers must appoint a "privacy officer" responsible for developing a program of compliance with HIPAA, conduct an assessment of privacy practices in the pharmacy, develop needed policies and procedures, and train employees on the regulation. HIPAA establishes penalties of up to 10 years in prison and $250,000 in fines for violations of the Act.

Conclusion

Now that you know how to prepare most prescriptions and to communicate with patients about them, you need to learn more details about the preparation of specialized prescriptions. In the next two chapters, we will consider the preparation, or compounding, of both nonsterile and sterile products for administration to patients.

For More Information

If you are preparing for the Pharmacy Technician Certification Examination and feel that you need more information about the topics discussed in this chapter, consider studying these sources of additional information:

- Berger BA. *Communication Skills for Pharmacists: Building Relationships, Improving Patient Care.* 2nd ed., a book published by APhA (available in the Store on www.pharmacist.com)
- The HIPAA information center on www.pharmacist.com
- Chapter 4 in the soon-to-be-published title from APhA, *The Pharmacy Technician's Introduction to Pharmacy,* by L. Michael Posey

TABLE 8-5

Cash in the Pharmacy

When handling cash, keep the following tips in mind:

- Follow to the letter all processes and procedures in your pharmacy about cash handling.

- Do not leave large bills outside the register while you count change. Most registers permit you to enter the amount of money the customer has given you, and the amount of change due is then displayed. This means there is no need for you to leave the money outside the register in an effort to remember how much you were given.

- If a customer seems to be trying to confuse you about money, stop and call on another pharmacy employee to listen and watch what you are doing so that you do not get "conned" by a swindler.

There is no acceptable reason to discuss outside your job anything that you learn while working as a pharmacy technician about people and the medications they are taking.

References

Ainsworth SR. Communications in pharmacy practice. In: Posey LM, ed. *Pharmacy Cadence 2002–2003*. Athens, GA: Pharmacy Editorial & News Services; 2002:29–36.

American Pharmacists Association. HIPAA information center. www.pharmacist.com/hipaa.cfm.

American Society of Health-System Pharmacists. ASHP guidelines on pharmacist-conducted patient education and counseling. *Am J Health Syst Pharm*. 1997;54:431–4.

Berger BA. *Communication Skills for Pharmacists: Building Relationships, Improving Patient Care*. 2nd ed. Washington, D.C.: American Pharmacists Association; 2005.

Latner AW. Pharmacy's HIPAA compliance deadline arrives. Accessed at http://www.pharmacist.com/articles/h_ts_0259.cfm, January 13, 2007.

Ranelli P. Patient communication. In: Gennaro RR, ed. *Remington: The Science and Practice of Pharmacy*. 19th ed. Easton, PA: Mack Publishing Company;1995:1779–85.

CHAPTER NINE

Nonsterile Compounding and Bulk Compounding

Chapter 9 briefly defines the process of compounding special prescriptions for patients. It then presents bulk compounding, along with regulatory distinctions between bulk compounding and manufacturing.

The process of mixing ingredients to prepare a special potion for a patient is compounding.

Compounding a prescription is a lot like baking a cake.

Introduction

Most medications needed on a daily basis in pharmacy practice are available in manufactured dosage forms. But pharmacists still frequently use their knowledge of medications and chemistry and their skills in the art of pharmacy to make special preparations—ones that would otherwise be unavailable—for patients. The process of mixing ingredients to prepare a special potion for a patient is *compounding*. As a technician, you may be called on to assist the pharmacist in compounding prescriptions for patients. Compounding occurs in all practice settings, including community, hospital, managed care, home care, and long-term care pharmacies, but is currently more common in independent and hospital pharmacies.

Nonsterile products are those intended to be used by mouth or externally (on the outside of the body). Examples include capsules, oral liquids, creams, ointments, emulsions, and pastes. Because these medications are placed into or on the body in places where natural defenses can stop any microorganisms that might be present, they do not need to be *sterile*, or free from bacteria, fungi, and viruses. This chapter describes the preparation of these nonsterile products. In addition, it details the preparation of large quantities of compounded products, called bulk compounding, along with specialized packaging machines that are used in pharmacy.

Equipment Used in Nonsterile Compounding

Compounding a prescription is a lot like baking a cake. You need to work in a clean, organized area; you work from a recipe or set of instructions; you need to gather all the right ingredients; you must accurately measure those ingredients and mix them in the correct order and manner; and you want the appearance of your final product to be pleasing. While the ingredients of prescriptions are very different, all these elements of baking apply to compounding.

For compounding, you need to learn how to use several basic types of equipment:

- **Weighing equipment** — By law, your pharmacy must have a prescription balance (Figure 9-1), that is, a scale used to weigh small quantities of solid or very thick semisolid pharmaceutical ingredients. Calibration of the scale is the first step in using it—check to make sure the balance has been zeroed, or calibrated, using procedures specific to that scale. Weighing papers (a type of waxed paper) or cups are used to keep ingredients from soiling or staining the pans on the scale. Other procedures used on scales vary, depending on the model and type. Ask your pharmacist to give you instructions on how to use the balance in your pharmacy. The most common scale present in pharmacies is a Class III balance. If you need to weigh quantities of less than 120 mg, this scale is not sufficiently accurate. Talk with the pharmacist to determine if a different type of scale is available for such small amounts. Scales must be calibrated periodically. This means that known quantities are measured on the scale to be sure the scale is accurate. Records should be kept of these calibrations as well as other equipment maintenance.

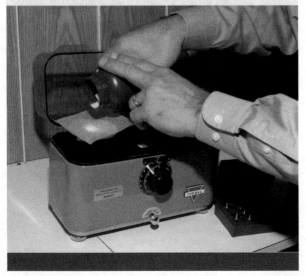

FIGURE 9-1

A prescription balance being used to weigh ingredients for compounding of a prescription.

• **Measuring equipment** — Your pharmacy should also be stocked with an appropriate supply of equipment for measuring liquids. For most nonsterile products, you will use a graduated cylinder to measure liquids. Several different sizes of these graduates should be available, such as 10 mL, 25 mL, 50 mL, 100 mL, and 1000 mL (Figure 9-2). So that your measurement is more accurate, you should select a graduate such that you are measuring an amount greater than 20% of its capacity. For instance, you would not measure 3 mL in a 100-mL graduate; rather you should use a 10-mL graduate. For measuring amounts of 0.1 mL to 5 mL, you may use syringes (without a needle attached). For very small amounts (less than 0.1 mL), micropipettes are used for measuring liquids.

• **Compounding equipment** — The pharmacy must also have an adequate supply of mortars and pestles (both glass, as shown in Figure 9-3, and Wedgwood or porcelain), stainless steel and plastic spatulas of different sizes, an ointment slab or pill tile, funnels, filter paper, beakers, glass stirring rods, a heat source (hot plate or microwave oven), a refrigerator, and a freezer. These are used in various steps of the compounding process, as directed.

• **Ingredients** — The pharmacist will generally stock the compounding area with chemicals that meet both the requirements of the *US Pharmacopeia and National Formulary* (USP/NF) and the Food and Drug Administration (FDA). USP/NF lists the standards the chemical must meet for strength, quality, and purity. FDA inspects the plants in which the chemicals were made for compliance with its "Good Manufacturing Practice" standards, ensuring that the chemicals are suitable for use in people. When selecting products for compounding, be sure that you pick the correct salt (for example, sodium chloride versus sodium phosphate) called for in the prescription. If you are crushing commercially available tablets to obtain a needed drug, do not use extended-release or delayed-release products.

Processes Used in Nonsterile Compounding

Many pharmaceutical ingredients can be mixed without any problems of compatibility. However, certain ingredients must be mixed carefully or in a special way to prevent problems in compounding. Pharmacists spend a considerable amount of time in college learning the principles and techniques used in these situations. While these principles and techniques cannot be detailed in this text, the following are brief descriptions of the basic techniques used most commonly to mix pharmaceutical ingredients:

• Trituration is a grinding of a drug solid using a mortar and pestle to reduce the particle size or to mix two or more solids (Figure 9-4). This technique is generally used to

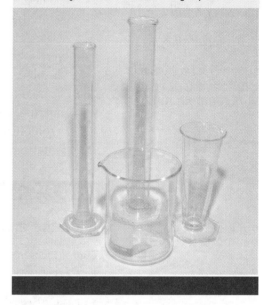

FIGURE 9-2

Graduated cylinders.

Graduated cylinders, the two taller containers shown in this photograph, should be used for measuring volumes of liquids in the pharmacy. The pharmaceutical graduate, shown on the right, can be used to measure liquids when accuracy is not as important, such as when an antibiotic suspension is being reconstituted. The beaker, shown in the front, should be used only for holding liquids, but it is not sufficiently accurate for measuring liquids.

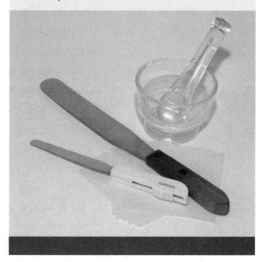

FIGURE 9-3

Other compounding elements.

Spatulas and a mortar and pestle, like the glass one shown here, are used in compounding. A mortar and pestle can also be made of porcelain; it is then called a Wedgwood mortar and pestle.

Many pharmaceutical ingredients can be mixed without any problems of compatibility. However, certain ingredients must be mixed carefully or in a special way to prevent problems in compounding.

(1) create a finer powder to make dissolution easier, (2) keep a cream or ointment from feeling gritty, or (3) ensure thorough mixing of solid ingredients.

- Levigation entails dispersing a drug solid in a small amount of mineral oil, glycerin, or other liquid before incorporating the paste into an ointment (often by trituration). This technique is used to keep the ointment from feeling gritty.

- Geometric dilution is used to ensure mixing of a small amount of a potent drug with a large amount of a nonpotent or inactive compound. The potent drug is triturated with an approximately equal amount of the other substance. That mixture is then combined with an approximately equal amount of the other substance, and so forth, until all of the second substance is incorporated.

- Sometimes it is necessary to increase dissolution. When preparing a solution, the solute (usually a solid drug) must be dissolved in the solvent (just like dissolving sugar or salt in water). Many drugs, being organic, carbon-based compounds, are not very soluble in water-based vehicles. That is, only a small amount of the drug will dissolve, or the substance dissolves very slowly. Various techniques can sometimes be used to increase the amount or rate of dissolution: heating the solvent or the mixture, reducing the particle size of the solute (by trituration or levigation), using a solubilizing agent that "coats" the solute and makes it dissolve more easily, or agitating the mixture by shaking or other means.

After the prescription has been compounded, inspect it for problems or signs of instability. These include particles in products that should be clear solutions, separation of ingredients in an emulsion or ointment, or discoloration on the outside of capsules. Based on your past experience or knowledge of what the product should look like, consult with the pharmacist if anything

TABLE 9-1

Choosing a Container

Considerations in choosing a container for a product include the following:

- Containers should meet specifications as described in the USP/NF and should be child-resistant unless the patient requests a non–child-resistant closure.

- To avoid medication errors, oral liquids should never be placed in syringes that can be used for injection (oral syringes—ones that will not accommodate a needle—are preferred).

- The container should not physically or chemically interact with the product.

- Amber or light-resistant containers should be used when the product is sensitive to light.

- The container should be of an appropriate size: The product should fill most or all of the container, and the container should hold all of the product.

FIGURE 9-4

A solid drug is being triturated, or ground into a smaller particle size, in this glass mortar and pestle.

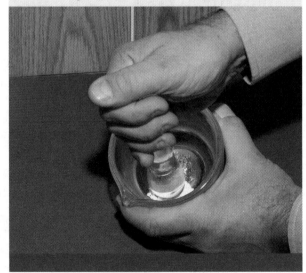

is not correct when you have finished mixing the ingredients. A properly prepared prescription should be pharmaceutically elegant: it should have the appropriate color, texture, smell, and feel when applied or used.

If the product appears to be correct and stable, you should place it in an appropriate container, as described in Table 9-1.

The final product must be labeled in accordance with state and federal laws, as shown in Table 9-2.

Some commonly used products may have acquired short names (for example, a pediatrician's product for diaper rash may be known locally by that physician's name, as in Smith's Goop). Labeling of product with such names is discouraged because the contents cannot be easily determined if a poisoning occurs. In addition, in instances where commercially available product has been used as the source of active ingredient in the prescription, the use of trade names is discouraged because the brand-name product has been altered in compounding the prescription.

The *beyond-use date* or *expiration date* is usually very short (not very far into the future) because compounded prescriptions are meant for immediate dispensing and use by the patient. The expiration date is assigned by the pharmacist after considering factors such as the following:

- Chemical stability: how long the chemicals as mixed are stable in each other's presence
- Physical stability: how long the product as mixed will remain in the proper form
- Microbial contamination: whether there is a risk of microbial growth in the product

An important element of compounding is keeping a record of the chemicals used in making each prescription. This record, while differing among pharmacies, usually includes the items listed in Table 9-3.

These records are critical in situations where a patient has an adverse reaction to a compounded product or when one of the ingredients is recalled by its manufacturer.

Bulk Compounding

When one or more prescribers in an area use the same compounded prescription repeatedly, pharmacists will sometimes make batches of the product to use when prescriptions are received. This process is called bulk compounding. It saves time for both the pharmacy and the patient, because many compounded prescriptions are complicated and patients typically would have to wait for them to be made.

During bulk compounding, an appropriate amount of product should be prepared based on the stability of the product and how often it is prescribed. After preparation, batches of product should be assayed for consistent potency (when applicable), tested for bacterial or other microbial growth (when applicable), and inspected routinely during storage for product instability, contamination, or breakdown.

TABLE 9-2

The Compounded Product Label

In addition to the elements required on labels of all prescriptions, the compounded product label should state:

- The generic or chemical name of all active ingredients
- Names of vehicles (the liquid used to make a solution or the ointment base used in compounding a topical product) if the vehicle differs among products (as when one vehicle contains sugar and another is sugar-free)
- Strength and/or quantity
- Pharmacy lot number (if applicable; see next section on Bulk Compounding)
- Beyond-use date
- Special storage requirements, if any

TABLE 9-3

Record of Chemicals in Prescriptions

The record of the chemicals used in making each prescription usually includes:

- Who prepared the product
- Names, manufacturers, lot numbers, and quantities of all ingredients used
- Order of mixing and special processes used
- Storage information
- Pharmacy lot number when a supply of product is made for several patients

In addition, the FDA has attempted to control how bulk-compounded products can be used, but its success at doing so has been mixed. FDA regulates manufacturers of drug products, such as big drug companies that conduct business across state lines, and pharmacies are for the most part regulated by state boards of pharmacy. This division works fine as long as pharmacies are clearly serving individual patients who, without prompting or advertising by the pharmacy, come in with a prescription that requires compounding. However, when pharmacies engage in bulk compounding, just where compounding ends and manufacturing begins is open to interpretation and discussion. In one case, the U.S. Supreme Court ruled that FDA bans on pharmacy advertising of compounded prescriptions and services was unconstitutional; hence, pharmacies can now advertise the availability of such services. The US Congress has held hearings on compounding, but no new laws have been passed clarifying the situation. Newspapers as prominent as the *Wall Street Journal* have run major articles assessing the legality, appropriateness, and logistics of the growing compounding business. FDA currently relies on a guidance it issued after its defeat in the US Supreme Court. The guidance lists nine criteria for deciding whether a facility should be investigated for possible violations. These include pharmacies that are compounding products in advance of prescriptions being presented for them, using medications that have been withdrawn from the US market for safety reasons, and using bulk active ingredients that are not approved by FDA. Another criterion states that with some exceptions, compounded products should not be duplicates of commercially available products or of FDA-approved drug products.

Pharmacists who might be pushing the envelope with regard to compounding services must turn to this FDA guidance in an effort to identify the line between legal and problematic practices. However, the guidance has been challenged by pharmacies in the federal courts, and this advice too could be struck down if it oversteps FDA's legal mandate as defined in the laws passed by Congress and signed by the President.

Repackaging

Many pharmacies are now repackaging commercially available drug products to fit into their automated dispensing machines and specialized drug-delivery systems. You may be involved in placing individual doses of medication into various types of strip packaging, pouch or blister cards (such as those shown in Figure 5-16), or oral syringes.

Blister cards are generally used in long-term care facilities (nursing homes, skilled-nursing facilities, intermediate-care facilities, assisted-living facilities) to help staff manage the medications that residents are taking. Similar cards with bigger bubbles, called pouch cards, are used to group all the tablets and capsules a patient takes at certain times of day; such packaging can help some patients (such as older patients who must take several medications each day) adhere to the therapies as prescribed and thereby avoid the need for institutionalization in long-term care facilities.

Repackaging of oral liquids usually involves oral syringes or cups. Never use syringes that can be used for injection to repackage oral liquids—nurses, patients, and others have injected these liquids, with sometimes fatal results. Also, because it is impossible to tell

TABLE 9-4

Repackaging Drug Products

Principles to keep in mind when repackaging products include:

- **Preparation:** Gather the correct drug products and supplies needed and organize them in a clean, neat work area.
- **Procedure:** Follow procedures carefully in using repackaging equipment in your pharmacy.
- **Quality control:** Check the repackaged product to be sure that everything is correct and that the drug product has not been damaged during the process.
- **Record keeping:** Record lot numbers of products used and other details meticulously in case questions arise, patients have adverse effects, or manufacturers recall the product.

what is in a liquid once it is repackaged, be extremely careful that you have the correct drug product and are placing the correct volume into the syringe or cup.

While the specifics of repackaging will depend on the type of equipment used in your pharmacy, the principles are the same as with compounding and bulk compounding, as shown in Table 9-4.

Conclusion

For some patients, the preparation of specially compounded prescription products is key to preventing or controlling disease. By carefully preparing pharmaceutically elegant compounded products, you can make an important difference in these patients' lives.

Many of the same principles you have learned in this chapter apply to the preparation of sterile products, which is the subject of Chapter 10. Let's take a look.

For More Information

If you are preparing for the Pharmacy Technician Certification Examination and feel that you need more information about the topics discussed in this chapter, consider studying these sources of additional information:

- Allen LV Jr. *The Art, Science, and Technology of Pharmaceutical Compounding*. 2nd ed. Washington, D.C.: American Pharmacists Association; 2002.
- Trissel LA. *Trissel's Stability of Compounded Formulations*. 3rd ed. Washington, D.C.: American Pharmacists Association; 2005.
- Moss Marks S, Hopkins WA Jr. *Pharmacy Technician Certification Quick-Study Guide*. 3rd edition. Washington, D.C.: American Pharmacists Association; 2006.

Reference

American Society of Hospital Pharmacists. ASHP technical assistance bulletin on compounding nonsterile products in pharmacies. *Am J Hosp Pharm*. 1994;51:1441–8. Available online at www.ashp.org/s_ashp/bin.asp?CID=6&DID=5462&DOC=FILE.PDF

During bulk compounding, an appropriate amount of product should be prepared based on the stability of the product and how often it is prescribed.

For some patients, the preparation of specially compounded prescription products is key to preventing or controlling disease.

CHAPTER TEN

Sterile Compounding and Radiopharmaceuticals

Chapter 10 highlights the basics of injectable-drug preparation. It presents topics such as sterile admixture, laminar flow, and aseptic technique to make the technician comfortable with these subject areas. Chapter 10 also presents radiopharmaceuticals in a concise format.

Many pharmacy technicians— especially in hospital, home care, and long-term care pharmacies but also in a growing number of community pharmacies—spend the majority of their time preparing sterile pharmaceutical products that are injected into patients.

Introduction

Many pharmacy technicians—especially in hospital, home care, and long-term care pharmacies but also in a growing number of community pharmacies—spend the majority of their time preparing sterile pharmaceutical products that are injected into patients. This is a specialized type of compounding, and the same principles and considerations apply to sterile products as were described in Chapter 9 for nonsterile preparations. The main difference is that you must make a special effort to avoid contamination of sterile products with microorganisms such as bacteria and fungi.

Some well-trained pharmacy technicians are hired directly into sterile-product—or intravenous admixture—positions. Others are promoted into such jobs after becoming familiar with medications and pharmacy practice through on-the-job experience in prescription or order filling or nonsterile compounding jobs. Some specialized pharmacies produce radiopharmaceuticals. These are prepared similarly to other sterile products, and some technicians work in this setting.

This chapter presents an overview of sterile product preparation for those technicians who have not yet trained or worked in this part of pharmacy practice. If you are already working in this area, you will need to consult more detailed manuals, training films, and educational materials, such as those listed at the end of this chapter, to increase your skills and knowledge about compounded sterile preparations (CSPs).

Aseptic Technique and Infection Control

In every step of the process of making CSPs, you must make a special effort to keep the preparation free of microbial growth. Microbes include the following organisms (Figure 10-1), ranked by size:

- Fungi
- Bacteria
- Viruses

Fungi are the largest of these microorganisms. Bread mold is an example of a fungus. When fungi are present in IV fluids, they may cause a moldlike growth in the solution, or they may simply make the fluid look cloudy. However, many millions of fungi and other microbes can be present in each milliliter of fluid without any visible changes.

Bacteria are the most common contaminants of IV fluids. They are large enough to be stopped by most filters used in admixture preparation or fluid administration to the patient. When they are present in large enough quantities (about 10 million to 100 million organisms per milliliter), the CSP will look cloudy or turbid.

Viruses are the smallest microbe. They are so small that they can pass through pharmaceutical filters. Viruses require a living host to grow, so they do not grow in IV fluids even though they may cause infection in the patient when the fluid is administered. They do not cause the solution to appear turbid, and they cannot be detected by commonly used methods of checking IV fluids for contamination. Thus, the patient's only defense against viruses is that they not be introduced into the fluid to begin with.

To avoid introducing microbial organisms into CSPs, pharmacists and technicians use aseptic technique in handling those products. Aseptic technique involves the taking of several precautions to prevent introduction of microbes into the products, including initial cleaning of the area used for manipulation of the products, creation of a sterile area and minimization of traffic in that area, gowning and gloving of the people working in the area, and quality controls to make sure that the procedures are in fact preventing contamination of the admixtures being produced. Before we look at what those procedures are, let's look at the many types of CSPs that are produced in pharmacies.

FIGURE 10-1

Examples of Microbes.

FIGURE 10-2

Intravenous Lines.

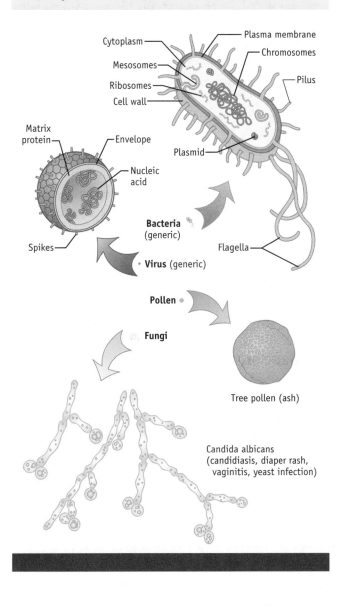

Cytoplasm
Plasma membrane
Chromosomes
Mesosomes
Ribosomes
Pilus
Cell wall
Matrix protein
Envelope
Plasmid
Nucleic acid
Bacteria (generic)
Spikes
Flagella
Virus (generic)
Pollen
Fungi
Tree pollen (ash)
Candida albicans (candidiasis, diaper rash, vaginitis, yeast infection)

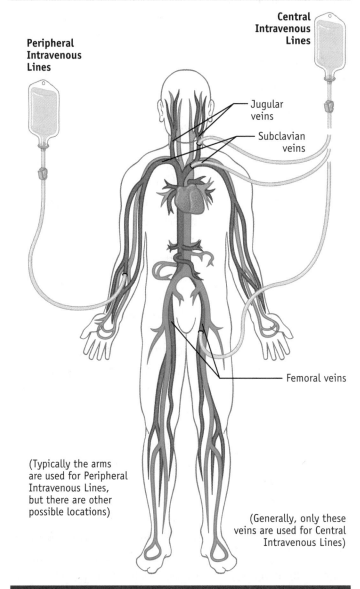

Central Intravenous Lines
Peripheral Intravenous Lines
Jugular veins
Subclavian veins
Femoral veins
(Typically the arms are used for Peripheral Intravenous Lines, but there are other possible locations)
(Generally, only these veins are used for Central Intravenous Lines)

Injectable Products

Because many CSPs are placed into patients' veins, they are often referred to generally as intravenous (or IV) fluids (Figure 10-2). For IV administration, the amount of fluid that is infused can vary considerably, but it is usually at least 50 mL to 100 mL and can range up to several liters of fluid per day. Other types of CSPs can be infused into arteries, administered into the fluid that surrounds the brain and spine, placed into the peritoneal cavity that surrounds the gastrointestinal organs of the gut, or placed into the eyes or joints of the body. CSPs are also used as baths for live organs and tissues after they are harvested from donors but before they are placed into recipients.

If the amount of IV fluid is less than 250 mL, it is a small-volume parenteral (SVP) solution. The main use of SVPs is for administering IV drugs to patients. For instance, a physician might order cefazolin 1 g IV every 8 hours for a patient with an infection. The pharmacy would prepare this amount of drug in 50 mL to 100 mL of a small-volume product, usually either 5% dextrose (a sugar solution) or 0.9% sodium chloride (a salt solution). These solutions would then be infused directly into the patient's veins.

To avoid introducing microbial organisms into CSPs, pharmacists and technicians use aseptic technique in handling those products.

SVPs are increasingly provided by manufacturers in a ready-to-infuse form. Some of these products are premixed solutions that are stored frozen until ready for use, while others keep the drug separate from the fluids until the time of dispensing or administration. Some newer products allow the drug and solution to be mixed in a closed system, and this is advantageous because the manipulation can safely occur in any location, even in the patient's home if needed. Ask someone in your pharmacy to show you the kinds of SVPs currently in use.

When larger amounts of IV fluids are required, the product is called a large-volume parenteral (LVP) solution. These are usually given to patients continuously, as in an order for 5% dextrose injection 125 mL/hr. In this case, the solution would keep running into the patient's veins during all hours of the day and night. The patient would receive 3 L/day of 5% dextrose injection (125 mL/hr × 24 hr), a common amount of IV fluid. When a patient has a "line" running continuously, the small-volume products are "piggybacked" onto that line, thereby decreasing the number of times a patient has to endure the discomfort of a venipuncture.

In addition to different sizes, IV fluids may be packaged in several different types of glass bottles, plastic bags, or plastic semirigid bottles. Generally within one hospital, health system, or community pharmacy, only one company's products are used. You should become familiar with those used in your work setting, including the various sizes and container types.

Special Considerations: Nutritional Solutions

In addition to SVPs used for drug delivery and LVPs used for volume replacement, pharmacies commonly produce specialized solutions. TPN is an important type of specialized solution that provides nutrition without the use of the gastrointestinal tract (hence the "parenteral," which means "other than enteral"). TPNs are used in clinical situations where patients cannot take any food or products by mouth, such as when surgery has been performed on the gastrointestinal tract and it needs to rest so that it can heal.

TPN solutions have high concentrations of glucose (up to 35%), amino acids, and sometimes fats. These solutions are so strong, or concentrated, that they would cause the patient problems if they were infused into a small vein. For this reason, most TPN solutions are administered through tubes inserted into a vein just before it reaches the heart (called central lines). However, some less-concentrated TPN solutions are infused into veins in the arms (peripheral lines). Peripheral lines are used in children, for adult patients who need only a few days of TPN, or in other specific clinical situations.

Any time that the needle of an IV administration set is inserted into a patient, there is an increased risk for infection because the skin—the body's first line of defense—is broken. This is true for peripheral lines, but it is even more critical for central lines because they are used for long time periods (weeks or months).

When TPN solutions are made in the pharmacy, the pharmacist or technician mixes concentrated glucose and amino acids to create the proper final amounts. Various electrolytes are added to the TPN solution, including sodium, potassium, acetate, chloride, magnesium, and calcium. Because calcium can form insoluble salts with some ingredients (such as phosphate), it must be added in a specific manner to prevent problems. Smaller amounts of vitamins, trace elements (such as chromium, copper, zinc, iodine, and manganese), and other ingredients are sometimes added according to the physician's instructions. Adult patients generally need about 2 L to 3 L/day of TPN solutions.

To assist in the preparation of TPN solutions, many pharmacies have a machine that can be programmed to mix the proper amounts of glucose, amino acids, and other solutions. These TPN compounders are computer-based machines that assist in calculations and help to keep the final products free of microbial contaminants. Some compounders can also add electrolytes, vitamins, and other ingredients based on your instructions. You need to keep two factors in mind when using a compounder, as discussed in Table 10-1.

If TPN is the only nutritional source for more than a couple of weeks, the patient will also need a source of fats. These are provided using commercially available emulsified fat products. They are sometimes administered separately because they can be administered via a peripheral line, or they can be mixed with the glucose–TPN solutions in a 3-in-1 admixture.

Another specialized nutritional product is enteral nutrition. These are liquid emulsions (similar in appearance to a milk shake) that are given through a tube inserted through the mouth or nose into the patient's stomach or small intestine. If at all possible, enteral nutrition solutions are used rather than TPN because they keep the patient's gastrointestinal tract active and avoid the need for an IV line going into a central vein. Some pharmacies handle enteral nutrition products, but they are also provided by dietitians, or, in some institutions, the dietary department.

Making Sterile Products in the Pharmacy

Until recently, the specific procedures used in pharmacy admixture preparation areas were determined mostly by the pharmacists in charge of that facility. In 2004, the United States Pharmacopeia (USP) finalized its General Chapter <797>, Pharmaceutical Compounding—Sterile Preparations. This document, which has the force of law because USP is recognized as a standards-setting organization in federal statutes and regulations, has created more uniform requirements and procedures.

To quote from the chapter, these USP standards "apply to all persons who prepare CSPs and all places where CSPs are prepared, e.g., hospitals and other health-care institutions, patient treatment clinics, pharmacies, physicians' practice facilities, and other locations and facilities in which CSPs are prepared, stored, and transported. Persons who perform sterile compounding include pharmacists, nurses, pharmacy technicians, and physicians. These terms recognize both that most sterile compounding is performed by or under the supervision of pharmacists in pharmacies and that this chapter applies to all healthcare personnel who prepare, store, and transport CSPs." At the time the second edition of this book was written, USP had issued several revisions to Chapter <797> and had collected comments from interested parties, but the finalized chapter had not been issued. Thus, the material presented here reflects the original 2004 version unless otherwise noted.

Chapter <797> provides practice and quality standards designed to prevent patient harm that could result from microbial, chemical, or physical contamination of CSPs or from preparation of CSPs that do not contain the right medications and fluids in the right amounts. The chapter also refers to CSPs with "excessive bacterial endotoxins." Endotoxins can end up in CSPs when bacteria have been introduced and then are burst, or lyse, because of the differences between the fluids and the organism's preferred environment. While the bacteria are dead, pieces of their cell walls and membranes and cellular structures remain in solution, and these can cause fever and other types of reactions when infused into patients. For this reason, USP specifies tests for endotoxins, which are also known as pyrogens, and you may hear pharmacists talking about these.

> **TABLE 10-1**
>
> ## Using a Compounder
>
> When using a compounder in the pharmacy, you must be aware of the following:
>
> The compounder must be properly calibrated, or adjusted, before you begin, and the proper solutions must be connected to the correct tubing as it goes through the compounder.
>
> Any error you make in entering the ingredients will result in the wrong product. These solutions are very concentrated, and errors can easily cause clinical problems in patients. Be very careful when entering the amounts of the ingredients. (To help prevent problems, many pharmacies require that two people check all TPN orders, calculations, and entries. Even if your pharmacy does not require this check, it is a good idea to ask a pharmacist or another knowledgeable technician to check your work when making TPN solutions.)

Persons who perform sterile compounding include pharmacists, nurses, pharmacy technicians, and physicians.

TABLE 10-2

Definitions and Examples of USP Chapter <797> Levels of Risk

VARIABLES	LOW RISK	MEDIUM RISK	HIGH RISK
Definition	CSPs are compounded within a physical area that restricts particle counts to 3,520 per square meter or less (referred to as ISO Class 5 or worse; in the past, this was referred to as a Class 100 environment); involve only the transfer, measuring, and mixing of closed or sealed packaging systems; manipulations are limited to opening ampuls, penetrating sterile stoppers on vials with sterile needles and syringes, and transferring sterile liquids in sterile syringes and sterile administration devices.	Multiple individual or small doses of sterile products are combined or pooled to prepare a CSP that will be administered either to multiple patients or to one patient on multiple occasions; the compounding process includes complex aseptic manipulations other than the single-volume transfer; and the compounding process requires unusually long duration.	CSPs include nonsterile ingredients, including manufactured products for nonsterile routes of administration or a nonsterile device is employed before the finished CSP is sterilized; or the CSP is made from sterile ingredients, components, devices, and mixtures that have been exposed to air quality inferior to ISO Class 5 (see definition in low-risk column of this table), including storage in such environments of opened or partially used packages of manufactured sterile products that do not contain antimicrobial preservatives.
Examples	Preparing admixtures using vials, ampuls, bottles, and bags whose contents are already sterile; making admixtures of not more than three manufactured products (including the infusion or diluent solution).	CSPs, such as TPN, made from multiple sterile products; adding or transferring drugs from multiple (defined as more than three in the proposed revision to <797>) vials or ampuls.	Dissolving nonsterile bulk drug and nutrient powders in solutions that are sterilized later; measuring and/or mixing sterile ingredients in nonsterile containers before later sterilization; assuming that bulk packages contain correct amounts of labeled active ingredients without verification that the product has not been adulterated or contaminated between uses.

Allowed beyond-use dating[a]

VARIABLES	LOW RISK	MEDIUM RISK	HIGH RISK
Room temperature	48 hours	30 hours	24 hours
Refrigeration	14 days	9 days	3 days
Frozen	45 days	9 days	3 days
Quality assurance requirements	Routine disinfection and air quality testing of compounding environment; visual confirmation that compounding personnel are properly wearing protective garb; review of all orders and packages for accuracy; visual inspection of CSPs for particulate matter, leakage, and accuracy and thoroughness of labeling.	Same as for low risk but with more challenging tests that are sometimes conducted more frequently than once a year.	Same as for low risk but with more challenging tests that are sometimes conducted at least twice a year.
Media-fill test procedures	Annual tests of each person authorized to work in area by having them manipulate vials and syringes containing bacterial growth broths, which are then incubated and inspected for bacterial growth.	Tests that are more challenging than for low risk and that are when appropriate conducted more frequently.	Tests involving preparation of bacterial growth media and use of positive controls, that are conducted at least twice a year.

[a] Time periods can be extended if sterility tests show CSPs are not contaminated.

Source: United States Pharmacopeia, Chapter <797>.

To increase the likelihood that patients receive unadulterated CSPs containing the right ingredients and fluids, Chapter <797> spells out requirements for sterile compounding policies and procedures, personnel training and evaluation, environmental quality and control, equipment used in CSP production, verification of automated procedures such as the TPN compounder described in the previous section, checks of finished products, storage and beyond-use (expiration) dating, quality control, packaging and transport/shipping of CSPs, patient or caregiver training, patient monitoring and adverse event reporting, and quality assurance programs. While discussion of all of these aspects is beyond the scope of this chapter, some basic aspects are described.

The USP Chapter <797> defines as its foundation the determination of whether personnel in the pharmacy, nursing station, or physician office are preparing CSPs with a low, medium, or high risk of microbial, physical, or chemical contamination. As shown in Table 10-2, USP defines these areas based on the types of products being used, the complexity of manipulations, and the quality of the environment in which compounding is conducted.

In the revised <797> that is in the works, a fourth category is defined, that of CSPs being prepared for immediate use. If adopted as it was described in the proposed revision, this category would exempt from the requirements of this chapter CSPs consisting of not more than three ingredients (including the solution or diluent) being prepared for emer-

FIGURE 10-3

Pharmacist working at a laminar-flow hood.

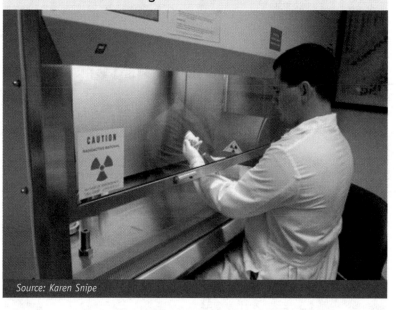

Source: Karen Snipe

FIGURE 10-4

Clean room.

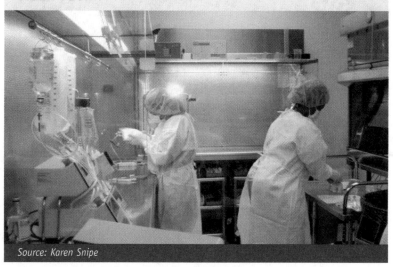

Source: Karen Snipe

gency or immediate (within 1 hour from the start of preparing the product) patient care. Immediate-use CSPs should be discarded if not used in 1 hour, the proposed language adds.

The physical environment set forth in USP Chapter <797> can be as simple as a laminar airflow cabinet or biological safety cabinet or as complex as a cleanroom, buffer zone, and anteroom. Laminar airflow hoods blow the air across the work surface in an even, or laminar, manner. Figure 10-3 illustrates aseptic technique in a horizontal laminar-flow hood. The vertical-flow biological-safety cabinet is discussed below in the section Special Considerations: Chemotherapy and Personal Protection.

In hospital pharmacies and other places making a lot of CSPs, cleanrooms are being built in response to USP Chapter <797> (Figure 10-4). These provide a large area meeting particulate requirements, and they generally have high-efficiency particulate air (HEPA)–filters that prevent microorganisms and particulate matter from entering the

FIGURE 10-5

Clean room attire.

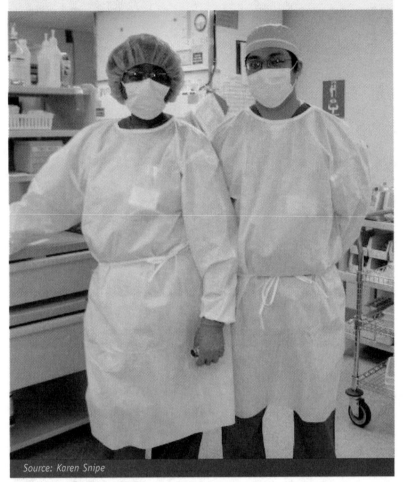

Source: Karen Snipe

TABLE 10-3

Quality Assurance of Sterile Products

When dealing with sterile products, quality assurance steps should include the following:

- Visual examination of the solution using a bright light placed behind the product (this helps to see particulate matter or precipitates)

- Sampling of the contents of products to measure key ingredients, such as a drug, sodium, potassium, chloride, or glucose (sugar)

- Sampling of the contents of selected products for microbial contamination

cleanroom. A buffer zone just outside the cleanroom is accessible only to staff authorized to work in the cleanroom, and only materials needed to make CSPs should be brought into the buffer zone.

Outside the buffer zone is an anteroom. Equipment not essential to making CSPs, such as computer stations or carts, can be placed outside the room in anterooms, but their effect on the environmental quality must be determined through testing and monitoring. Anterooms may contain sinks and drains (these are not permitted in the buffer zone or cleanroom), and anterooms provide places for personnel to scrub their hands and arms and put on the special clothes worn to prevent CSP contamination.

Personnel working in IV admixture areas should wear gloves while handling products to avoid introducing organisms present on the skin or under the fingernails into the product and gowns, masks, and shoe and hair covers like those used in operating rooms, to prevent microorganisms on their clothes from being introduced into the clean area. Goggles are sometimes worn, but these are more to protect the eyes from spills and sprays of the medications being manipulated, as discussed in the next section. The gloves, gowns, masks, shoe and hair covers, and goggles are collectively called protective garb (Figure 10-5).

The proposed revisions to Chapter <797> provide detailed guidelines for appropriate personal grooming for those working in clean areas. Personnel working in CSP preparation areas must keep their nails trimmed neatly (artificial nails and extenders are prohibited) and should remove all cosmetics (since they can shed flakes and particles), outside garments such as bandannas, coats, hats, and jackets, and all hand, wrist, or body jewelry (including visible body piercings above the neck) before entering the clean area.

Food, drinks, candy, and chewing gum are not permitted in any of the three clean areas.

Detailed standard operating procedures for the cleanroom are suggested in the USP Chapter <797>. Some general concepts are described here. Within a laminar airflow hood, the sterile air is usually flowing from the back toward the front, where the operator stands. The hood should be cleaned and disinfected with an agent such as isopropyl alcohol at the beginning of each shift, or more frequently if needed. To keep the product free from contamination, never put your hands or nonsterile equipment between the flow of air and the product. Use alcohol wipes to disinfect the tops of vials or the entry ports on containers before you puncture them with needles. After removing them from the protective packaging, handle the syringes and needles in such a way that you never place your hands or nonsterile equipment between them and the flow of sterile air. By using aseptic technique properly, you minimize the chances of introducing microbes into the sterile product.

Materials used in making CSPs must generally be discarded as biomedical waste. Follow the procedures in your pharmacy or institution to comply with applicable laws and regulations.

As with bulk compounding, you must make a special effort with sterile products to be certain that they have the correct ingredients, that the products are free from contamination, and that no precipitate (substances that are not dissolved into the solution) or particulate matter is in the bottle. Quality assurance steps with sterile products include those presented in Table 10-3.

The application of the quality assurance methods will be described further in Chapter 14.

In addition to these efforts to avoid introducing microorganisms into patients, hospitals and other health institutions make many other efforts to control infections in patients. Since the introduction of antibiotics in the middle of the 20th century, microorganisms have become increasingly resistant to their effects. Some bacteria and other microbes that can cause serious or fatal infections no longer respond to even the most powerful antibiotics. As a result, infection-control methods that prevent infection, eliminate sources of microbes, and avoid development of antibiotic resistance have become more and more important.

You may encounter infection-control measures such as those presented in Table 10-4.

Special Considerations: Chemotherapy and Personal Protection

A specialized type of IV product made in the pharmacy is the chemotherapy admixture. Generally used to treat cancer, chemotherapy drugs often require special handling or dilution. In addition, these powerful drugs can actually cause cancer (that is, they are *carcinogens*) because they disrupt the cycles of both normal and cancer cells. They also can cause birth defects (that is, they are also *teratogens*) or impair fertility, particularly in women of child-bearing age but also potentially in men.

Thus, it is important for the pharmacist or technician who is handling chemotherapy drugs (Figure 10-6) to take special precautions to keep the product off their own bodies (to prevent absorption through the skin) and out of their mouths, throat, and lungs (to prevent absorption through the mucous membranes). Four goals describe the efforts made in most pharmacies, institutions, and home care settings to prevent exposure to chemotherapy agents by workers (including pharmacy, nursing, delivery, and other personnel), patients, patients' families, and visitors. They are presented in Table 10-5.

TABLE 10-4

Measures to Control Infection

Infection-control measures that you may encounter in institutions and health systems include the following:

- Physical precautions require you to use special protective equipment when entering patients' rooms if they have certain infections or if they are easily susceptible to infection.
- Chemical precautions entail keeping all parts of the hospital clean and free of molds and mildew.
- Antibiotic restrictions limit the use of certain anti-infective agents to serious situations, thereby preventing the development of resistance in patients who could have used other agents.
- Decreases in the use of antibiotics for prevention and in situations where bacteria are not a likely or a known cause of infection (such as when people have the common cold) help to limit the development of antibiotic resistance.

FIGURE 10-6

Hospital pharmacy technician preparing a chemotherapy solution.

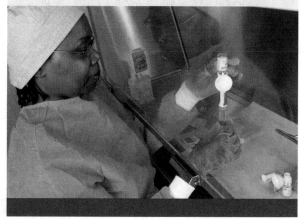

Preventing Exposure to Chemotherapy Agents

To prevent accidental exposure to chemotherapy agents, pharmacists should:

- Protect and secure packages of hazardous drugs.
- Inform and educate all involved personnel about hazardous drugs and train them in safe-handling procedures relevant to their responsibilities.
- Do not let drugs escape from containers when they are manipulated.
- Eliminate the possibility of inadvertent ingestion or inhalation and direct skin or eye contact with the drugs.

A specialized type of IV product made in the pharmacy is the chemotherapy admixture.

Pharmacies have instituted precautionary measures to help minimize the chance of exposure to hazardous substances. Some of them are described in Table 10-6. A barrier hood, sometimes used in chemotherapy preparation, is shown in Figure 10-7.

Radiopharmaceuticals

A few pharmacies specialize in handling radiopharmaceuticals, which are medications that contain radioactive compounds. These pharmacies are also called nuclear pharmacies.

To comprehend radioactivity and nuclear pharmacy, you need to recall a few definitions from chemistry:

- *Atoms* are the smallest particles in nature that still retain the characteristics of the substance from which they came. Atoms are made up of three subatomic particles: protons, neutrons, and electrons (see Figure 4-1).

Precautionary Measures with Hazardous Substances

Some of the ways pharmacies protect workers from accidental contamination with hazardous agents include:

- Warning labels are applied to packages containing chemotherapy drugs, and shipping boxes from manufacturers contain warning symbols.
- Sometimes biological safety cabinets are used to manipulate chemotherapy products. These cabinets use a vertical flow of air to prevent the materials being manipulated from blowing onto the pharmacist or technician.
- Pharmacists and technicians should always wear two sets of latex gloves ("double gloving"), and one or both sets of gloves should be discarded between products or batches or if the gloves are torn or punctured.
- A disposable gown should be worn to protect the body and clothes from contamination.
- Masks should be worn to prevent contamination of the respiratory tract, particularly if a biological safety cabinet is not being used. However, these masks provide no protection against powdered or liquid aerosols (very fine sprays) of these drugs.
- A plastic face shield or splash goggles should be worn if eye contact with the drugs is possible.
- Syringes and needles should have Luer-lock fittings to minimize the possibility of separation during product preparation. In addition, other devices may be used in your work setting, including safety needles, vented needles, filters, and filter needles. Be sure that you thoroughly understand such equipment before you use it.
- Needles should not be recapped after use to minimize needlestick injuries to workers. Syringes and needles should be disposed of as hazardous materials in accordance with the policies in your workplace (which must comply with federal, state, and sometimes local laws and regulations). After administering the admixture to a patient, nurses or other personnel should discard as hazardous materials the container, administration set, and other materials that might have come in contact with the chemotherapy drug.

- *Protons* are subatomic particles found in the nucleus (or middle) of an atom. The number of protons defines what substance the atom is, such as carbon, oxygen, or hydrogen. For instance, an atom with 6 protons is carbon, an atom with 8 protons is oxygen, and an atom with 1 proton is hydrogen. Protons have a positive charge.

- *Electrons* are very, very small subatomic particles that circle around the nucleus. You might think of the sun as the nucleus, with the planets circling around the sun like electrons. Electrons are so small that their weight is not considered when determining the mass of an atom. Because electrons carry a negative charge, a proton and an electron together are neutral.

- *Neutrons*, as their name implies, are neutral—they do not have a charge. They are located in the nucleus of the atom with the protons. An atom can have any number of neutrons without changing into another kind of atom, as long as the number of protons remains the same. For instance, carbon normally has 6 protons, 6 neutrons, and 6 electrons, and its total molecular weight is 12 (6 protons + 6 neutrons; the electrons do not count).

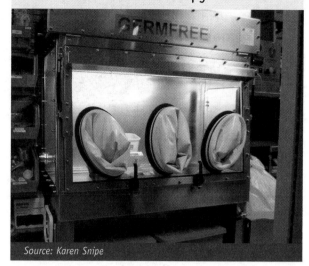

FIGURE 10-7

USP <797> chemotherapy hood.

Source: Karen Snipe

As long as the atom in the above example keeps the 6 protons, it will be carbon. It can have 6, 7, or 8 neutrons, and still be carbon, as long as it has 6 protons. When it has 7 neutrons, its molecular weight is 13, and the atom is called "carbon-13." When it has 8 neutrons, its molecular weight is 14, and it is called "carbon-14." All three of these are called isotopes of carbon.

Some isotopes are not stable because of the arrangement of the protons and neutrons in the very tight nucleus. These isotopes will decay over time and spontaneously transform into a more stable form. They decay by emitting particles from the neutrons, protons, or both. The particles are of three types: alpha particles, beta particles, and gamma particles. These particles can be detected by special instruments (such as Geiger counters or scintillation counters) and photographic films that are sensitive to specific radiation (such as x-ray film).

- *Alpha particles:* the emission of two protons and two neutrons from the nucleus into the environment. This changes the substance from one element to another (the one with two fewer protons).

- *Beta particles:* a neutron changes into a proton and an electron, and the proton stays in the nucleus and the electron is emitted into the environment. This changes the substance into the element with one more proton.

- *Gamma particles:* high-energy radiation that does not affect protons, neutrons, or electrons. This type of radiation, which approaches the power of X-rays, usually occurs with alpha and beta radiation.

To return to the carbon example above, carbon-14 is not as stable as the other isotopes of carbon. It will gradually, over thousands of years, return to a more stable form. It does so by emitting a beta particle and thereby changing into nitrogen-14. These emissions occur along very precise timelines that are described as the half-life of the isotope, that is, the amount of time required for one half of the atoms to change from the unstable to the stable state. For carbon-14, the half-life is 5,730 years. In the process of carbon dating, the half-life of carbon-14 is used to estimate the age of archaeological relics—those items dug up on the sites of ancient cities and civilizations.

You must make a special effort with sterile products to be certain that they have the correct ingredients, that the products are free from contamination, and that no precipitate (substances that are not dissolved into the solution) or particulate matter is in the bottle.

FIGURE 10-8

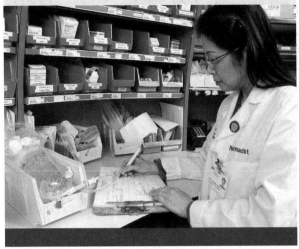

Hospital pharmacist performing a final check of a chemotherapy solution.

In nuclear medicine, the various properties of radioactive elements and compounds are used to detect, assess, and treat disease in people. Some examples of clinically useful radioisotopes include the following:

- *Iodine-131* is used to assess thyroid function and to treat thyroid overactivity and cancer.
- *Technetium-99m* is used in imaging many parts of the body. The "m" after the 99 stands for "metastable," which indicates that it does not change into another element after decay. It remains technetium-99 by emitting only gamma radiation. The half-life of this agent is only 6 hours, making it very useful in clinical imaging because it does not expose the patient to prolonged radiation.
- *Cobalt-60* is used in radiation therapy for cancer.

Because many of the radioisotopes used in medicine have short half-lives, nuclear pharmacists must generate the isotope and provide the preparation to the nuclear medicine department just before various imaging studies or treatments are to be performed. Radioisotope (also called radionuclide) generation is a daily procedure in the nuclear pharmacy. In situations where no nuclear pharmacy is available, nuclear medicine departments prepare radionuclides using commercially available kits.

All aspects of sterile compounding apply to nuclear pharmacy practice. In addition, other quality control considerations must be kept in mind, including checks required by the federal Nuclear Regulatory Commission:

- *Radionuclide purity* is the proportion of radioactivity that comes from the correct radioisotope. For instance, if the preparation is labeled as iodine-131, how much of the radioactivity present is actually generated by iodine-131?
- *Radiochemical purity* is the portion of the labeled radionuclide that is in the stated chemical form. For instance, if chromium-51 is in a solution of sodium chromate, how much of the radioactive chromium is in this chemical complex?
- *Specific activity* is the amount of radioactivity per unit weight of the compound. This is expressed in millicuries (mCi), a unit of radioactivity, per milligram of compound. Generally, this number should be as high as possible, but there are situations where more nonradioactive compound needs to be present for the radioactive compound to reach its active site.
- *Radioactivity concentration* is the amount of radioactivity (in mCi) per milliliter of solution. Again, high radioactivity concentrations are preferred.

Conclusion

Pharmacy technicians who have the necessary knowledge and skills make valuable contributions through their work in sterile product preparation. If the ideas and information in this chapter appeal to you, seek out more information from pharmacists you work with (Figure 10-8) or in the references listed below.

One aspect of the prescription process remains to be explored—how the pharmacy gets paid. That's the subject of Chapter 11.

For More Information

If you are preparing for the Pharmacy Technician Certification Examination and feel that you need more information about the topics discussed in this chapter, consider studying these sources of additional information:

- Snipe K. Sterile compounding. In: *The Pharmacy Technician Skills-Building Manual.* Washington, D.C.: American Pharmacists Association; 2007:107–28.
- United States Pharmacopeia. <797> Pharmaceutical compounding—sterile preparations [proposed revisions—redline version]. Rockville, Md.: United States Pharmacopeial Convention; 2006. Accessed at http://www.usp.org/pdf/EN/USPNF/PF797redline.pdf, January 14, 2007.
- ASHP Compounding Center, www.ashp.org, including the Self-Assessment Tool for Compounding Sterile Preparations, accessed at http://www.ashpbestpracticessat.com/797.html, January 14, 2007.
- Kostango ES, Bradshaw BD. USP chapter 797: establishing a practice standard for compounding sterile preparations in pharmacy. *Am J Health Syst Pharm.* 2004;61:1928–38. http://www.ajhp.org/cgi/reprint/61/18/1928.pdf.

References

United States Pharmacopeia. <797> Pharmaceutical compounding—sterile preparations [proposed revisions—redline version]. Rockville, Md.: United States Pharmacopeial Convention; 2006. Accessed at http://www.usp.org/pdf/EN/USPNF/PF797redline.pdf, January 14, 2007.

American Society of Health-System Pharmacists. ASHP guidelines on handling hazardous drugs. *Am J Health Syst Pharm.* 2006;63:1172–93. Accessed at http://www.ashp.org/s_ashp/bin.asp?CID=6&DID=5420&DOC=FILE.PDF, January 14, 2007.

CHAPTER ELEVEN

How Pharmacies Are Paid for Prescriptions

Chapter 11 highlights the key facts technicians need to know in assisting with billing for reimbursement. It includes descriptions of payment mechanisms, types of payers and intermediaries, and the importance of accuracy in data entry.

Most prescriptions
are paid for by
outside entities,
which are collectively
known as
third-party payers.

Introduction

Until the establishment of the Medicaid and Medicare programs in the 1960s, pharmacists charged individual patients for the prescription drugs they received. Since that time, however, the payment of pharmacies by governmental agencies, insurance companies, and health plans has become increasingly important. Today, most prescriptions are paid for by these outside entities, which are collectively known as *third-party payers*. With the launching of Medicare Part D in 2006 (see Chapter 3), nearly every prescription in many pharmacies are covered by some type of third-party plan.

This chapter describes the types of payers and special nuances about each. You can use this information to place in perspective those tasks you are asked to complete that help to ensure that your pharmacy gets paid for the products and services it provides.

Understanding the Methods of Payment

Pharmacists are generally paid for prescriptions in one of three ways:

- Direct payment by the patient
- Reimbursement from a governmental program, usually either Medicaid (for indigent patients) or Medicare (for the elderly and the disabled)
- Reimbursement from a nongovernmental payer, such as a managed care plan, insurance company, or employer

Let's consider some aspects of each of these three methods of payment.

Direct Payment

Patients whose health care or insurance plans do not cover prescription drugs must pay the pharmacy directly. Once the most common method of payment, direct payment has dramatically declined over the past couple of decades as health plans and now Medicare have added prescription drug coverage.

The decline of direct payment can be troublesome for independent community pharmacies. Patients who are paying for their own prescriptions are able to pick the pharmacy of their choice, making their selection based on the quality of professional services they receive. As will become clearer below, independent pharmacies are not always included in third-party networks, and patients can be forced to end long-standing relationships with their pharmacists when their prescription drug benefits are not available in that pharmacy.

In addition, pharmacies do not necessarily charge all direct-payment patients the same prices, even for the same drug products. Pharmacy computer systems have several different pricing schemes that the owner or managers can set up, and these result in different prices. Just as airlines charge passengers different prices for the same trip, pharmacists charge different amounts based on the services they provide. For instance, a patient who always charges prescriptions (to a store account) and has the medications delivered will likely pay higher prices. Someone who is very cost-conscious—perhaps who always wants the cheapest generic product or seems very concerned about medication costs—will likely be coded to receive lower prices. While this situation may sound inequitable, it is in fact the way many businesses operate—the owner sets prices based on the costs of the product and service, overhead, business strategies, and expected profit. If you have concerns about it or the specific situation in your pharmacy, talk with your pharmacist about how prescription drug prices are set in your pharmacy.

The decline of direct payment can be troublesome for independent community pharmacies.

Reimbursement by Governmental Agencies

The federal Centers for Medicare & Medicaid Services (CMS) manages the huge Medicare and Medicaid programs, which provide some $600 billion in reimbursements to health care providers (hospitals, physicians, pharmacies, and other types of health providers) each year. The Medicare program covers primarily acute care for the elderly, while the Medicaid program covers the indigent (people of all ages who have low, usually poverty-level, income and few assets). Medicare pays for prescription drugs if they are used in an acute-care institution (hospital) or if they are used in conjunction with certain medical devices such as in-dwelling catheters. Medicaid pays for outpatient prescription drugs (including those dispensed from community pharmacies) and other care in nursing homes or hospitals. Medicare Part D covers outpatient prescription drugs for the elderly and the disabled, and Part B covers certain injectable drugs.

Even though the Medicare and Medicaid systems are administered by CMS, they work very differently from one another. As was described in Chapter 3, Medicare Part D is administered through dozens of private prescription drug providers, or PDPs. Every PDP has its own formulary, and Medicare beneficiaries can choose any PDP operating in their geographic area (usually a state). Pharmacists' interactions are generally with these intermediaries when it comes to obtaining reimbursement for prescriptions and getting approval for nonformulary medications. Pharmacies must contract with these intermediaries, and either party can decline to contract with the other. Thus, the owner or managers of your pharmacy may have decided not participate in all plans available in your state or geographic region, or some PDPs may have declined to contract with your pharmacy (perhaps because few enrollees live in your area, the plan managers believed they had enough pharmacies available in the city or town, or the two parties simply could not agree on terms).

Medicaid works quite differently. Even though about one half of the money for Medicaid comes from CMS, the rest comes from state governments, which are directly responsible for their own Medicaid programs. These programs vary from state to state. Nearly all pharmacies are recognized Medicaid providers (making it an *open network*, rather than a *closed network*, which might be limited to a small number of pharmacies in a city or town). For a pharmacy to be recognized, its owner or manager must enter into a contract with the state Medicaid agency. The state agency will likely have many requirements, as shown in Table 11-1.

To get paid by third-party payers, including Medicare PDPs and Medicaid, the pharmacy must file claims for the prescriptions dispensed. Using Internet or modem-to-modem connections these claims are generally transmitted by the pharmacy computer system at the same time as prescriptions are dispensed by the pharmacy. This means that any error in the computer—whether patient name or plan number, National Drug Code number, incorrect quantity or directions—will result in either an incorrect payment to the pharmacy or a rejected claim. It can be very difficult to correct such mistakes once they occur. When entering any prescription into the computer, you must be very careful to get everything correct to avoid problems with both patients and reimbursement.

Third-party payers generally reimburse pharmacies for the cost of the drug plus a professional dispensing fee. In determining the cost of the drug, most state Medicaid programs differentiate between those medications that are available from multiple manufacturers (multisource products) and those that are available through only one company (single-source products). For a multisource product—regardless of how much the pharmacy paid and whether the name-brand or generic product was dispensed—Medicaid will generally pay only for the cheaper generic product. In some states, the Medicaid program has a list of

TABLE 11-1

State Agency Requirements for Medicaid

State agencies will likely have many requirements to enter into a contract with a pharmacy. They include:

- All Medicaid patients must be served without discrimination.

- The prices charged Medicaid must be equal to or lower than the best prices given any other payer or patient of the pharmacy.

- All Medicaid patients must be offered the opportunity to be counseled about their medications by the pharmacist.

- The pharmacy must review Medicaid prescriptions and identify improper or incorrect prescribing patterns and work with physicians to improve them.

Just as airlines charge passengers different prices for the same trip, pharmacists charge different amounts based on the services they provide.

When entering any prescription into the computer, you must be very careful to get everything correct to avoid problems with both patients and reimbursement.

frequently used multisource drug products for which it has established maximum allowable costs. For these products, Medicaid will pay only for the cheapest of the generic products.

In December 2006, CMS proposed new regulations that would pin pharmacy reimbursements on prescription drug prices posted to a publicly available Web site. If implemented as originally proposed, this could further constrict the amounts pharmacies are paid for prescriptions.

Medicare pays for hospitalized patients (inpatients) based on a set amount for various *diagnosis-related groups*, or *DRGs*. For instance, for a Medicare beneficiary with uncomplicated pneumonia, Medicare might pay $3,000 to the hospital, regardless of how long the patient stays in the institution or what drugs or procedures are performed. The incentive in such a system is for hospitals to provide more efficient care. However, some critics have denounced this *prospective-payment system* as encouraging hospitals to discharge elderly patients "sicker and quicker." In addition, CMS has been analyzing whether specialty hospitals are declining to accept transfers of patients with complicated illnesses from community hospitals, thereby allowing the specialty hospitals to profit from the less-sick patients within a given DRG and causing financial problems at the community hospitals (and placing the very patients who need more specialized care in danger).

If a Medicare patient receives unusually expensive care during a hospitalization, the institution may qualify for direct reimbursement outside the DRG system. Cost of care for these outliers is sometimes driven up by expensive medications, especially those derived from biotechnology research. When this is the case, pharmacy personnel are sometimes involved in determining those costs.

Third-party payers generally reimburse pharmacies for the cost of the drug plus a professional dispensing fee.

An area of much concern is fraud and abuse in the Medicaid and Medicare systems. This situation occurs when health care providers (most often physicians or dentists, but increasingly nurses or pharmacists) bill the government for products or services that were not provided to patients. Specific problems uncovered in pharmacy include the following:

- Billing for nonexistent prescriptions and for medications not dispensed
- "Partial filling," in which the pharmacy gives the patient part of the quantity called for in a legitimate prescription (asking the patient to come back later to get the rest) and bills Medicaid for the full quantity, but doesn't return part of the reimbursement if the patient never returns
- Billing for name-brand products when generic alternatives are actually dispensed

An area of much concern is fraud and abuse in the Medicaid and Medicare systems.

These problems are usually uncovered by either computer detection of unusual dispensing patterns in a given pharmacy or by whistleblowers, people who come forward with information about activity they believe to be fraudulent. During investigation of the problem, state Medicaid or other government officials likely will visit the pharmacy for an in-store audit. You might be asked to help them find records for prescriptions they are checking on. It is important that the pharmacy provide as much documentation of the validity of prescriptions as possible during such audits, which can be the last step before criminal prosecutions. (Note that Medicaid also conducts in-store audits as part of routine compliance checking. Do not assume that an audit means someone suspects a problem.)

Corporations have had to pay large fines in connection with fraud and abuse. Individual pharmacists have sometimes been convicted of fraud and have had to pay personal fines, serve prison time, or both. "Whistleblowers" sometimes share in these fines with the government if they have participated in the case in certain ways. Some individuals have been paid millions of dollars for uncovering extensive patterns of fraud and abuse.

Reimbursement by Nongovernmental Third-Party Payers

The Medicaid reimbursement model described above is fairly simple. In a given state, there is one payer, one set of rules, and one set of beneficiaries. The pharmacy receives the prescription order and dispenses the medication, and someone pays for it.

But when you add in Medicare Part D, the PDPs, and other nongovernmental third-party payers, the situation becomes exceedingly more complex. Patients are covered under many different policies and plans, each with its own rules and coverage limits. Drugs may be covered under one plan (by being on that plan's formulary, or preferred drug list) but may not be on the list of another plan (even one from the same company). The amount the patient must pay (copayment) differs between plans and for different types of medications (brand-name or generic products, formulary or nonformulary status).

Most patients whose prescription medications are covered under these plans are employees who receive prescription coverage as part of their benefits package at work. Several different entities are involved in such prescription drug benefits:

- **Employers** — Most large employers have very active human resource departments that manage employee benefits programs. Because health care is such an expensive employee benefit, it gets a lot of attention from human resource personnel. While it is not likely that you would contact the employer directly about a specific prescription, pharmacists and pharmacy owners sometimes meet with human resource personnel to talk about problems their policies are causing for the employees or to offer to provide additional services to a group of employees (such as diabetes care or smoking cessation for employees in a factory or asthma monitoring for employees or their children). Employers are very receptive to interventions that can increase employees' productivity by making them healthier or decreasing absences from work (including time off to care for sick children or take children to physician office visits).

- **Insurance companies** — Some employees choose traditional insurance companies for their coverage. In addition, most small employers and individuals who must purchase their own policies contract with insurance companies for health care coverage. These companies may have their own networks set up for care, or they may contract with some or all of the types of organizations listed below.

- **Managed care plans** — Employers may contract with *managed care plans* or organizations to provide health care benefits to covered workers and their families (collectively called *covered lives*). The employer pays a set amount into the plan each month per person or family, meaning that the income available to the managed care plan is a fixed amount per individual. For this reason, managed care plans base many of their financial analyses and projections on how much they are spending per person for each component of health care (for example, drugs, hospital care, doctor visits). These calculations can be *per member per month* (PMPM) or *per member per year* (PMPY). These plans are increasingly asking pharmacies to share in their risk by paying a fixed amount, such as $10 PMPM, regardless of the number of prescriptions dispensed.

- **In-house pharmacies** — Some managed care organizations are health-maintenance organizations (HMOs) that hire their own providers (physicians, nurses, pharmacists, technicians) and purchase their own facilities (care centers, hospitals, pharmacies). A prominent example of this type of staff-model HMO in many large US cities is Kaiser Permanente. In such plans, patients have a strong financial incentive to obtain their medications at these pharmacies: Copayments are lower at in-house pharmacies than at outside pharmacies.

Patients are covered under many different policies and plans, each with its own rules and coverage limits.

Because health care is such an expensive employee benefit, it gets a lot of attention from human resource personnel.

- **Third-party administrators** — Outside the staff-model HMO, other managed care plans contract for some or all of the services they offer. For the prescription drug benefit, these plans either contract with a *third-party administrator* (TPA) or a pharmacy benefits management company (see below). TPAs are companies that issue drug cards to beneficiaries, organize networks of pharmacy providers, and pay those pharmacies for the prescriptions they dispense to beneficiaries. These networks may be open (all pharmacies can become members) or closed (not all pharmacies are able to join). TPAs are paid a set fee per paid claim by the managed care plan—the more prescriptions are dispensed, the more the TPA is paid. Likewise, the TPA pays each pharmacy for the cost of the drug plus a dispensing fee, with increased prescriptions meaning increased revenues to the pharmacy.

- **Pharmacy benefits managers** — Reimbursement for prescriptions is often handled through an intermediary company, such as PCS Health Systems or Medco. These companies, known as *pharmacy benefits managers*, or PBMs, are very important parts of the current payment system in community pharmacy. PBMs differ from TPAs in that they are more involved in clinical activities and programs such as patterns of drug use among prescribers, pharmacies, and groups of patients; establishment and enforcement of preferred drugs as listed in formularies; disease management; prior authorization of selected or expensive drugs; and establishment of prescribing guidelines. PBMs are typically involved in payments for Medicare Part D prescriptions, acting as an intermediary between the PDPs and pharmacies. While some PBMs are paid by plans for each prescription processed, they are increasingly paid a set amount PMPM. For instance, a plan might pay to the PBM a fee of $10 PMPM for all drugs needed by members of the plan. This puts the PBM at risk with the plan, especially because most pharmacies are still reimbursed for each prescription processed. This capitated arrangement—payment of a fixed amount of money per person—gives the PBM an incentive to ensure efficiency in care and to reduce the use of unnecessary drugs or expensive agents for which cheaper alternatives would be just as good. PBMs may also require that patients get long-term supplies of medications for chronic diseases from PBM-owned mail-service pharmacies, which dispense several months' supply of medications from warehouse locations in other states and send it to the patient via the US mail or an overnight delivery service.

Depending on the kind of pharmacy you work in, you may see these entities from very different perspectives. But regardless of where you are, you can be sure that they are increasingly important in pharmacy and the overall health care system.

TABLE 11-2

The Point-of-Service System

The point-of-service system enables the pharmacy to perform the following functions at the time a prescription is dispensed:

- Verify eligibility of the beneficiary for prescription benefits
- Determine that the medication is covered
- Obtain prior authorization of restricted medications
- Determine the maximum quantity that may be dispensed and whether there is a maximum allowable cost for multisource products
- For a refill of an older prescription, make sure it is not being refilled too early
- Check for possible drug–drug interactions
- Confirm the amount of copayment
- Submit the claim for payment

TABLE 11-3

CPT Codes Used Most Frequently by Pharmacists for New Patients and Initial Consultations

CODE	LEVEL	HISTORY	DECISION	EXAMPLES	TIME
99201	level 1	problem-focused	straightforward	review basics of oral agent/insulin with patient who has been on agent in past	10 min
99202	level 2	expanded problem-focused	straightforward	complete education provided for the patient receiving oral agent/insulin for the first time	20 min
99203	level 3	detailed	low complexity	complete education of oral agent/insulin and evaluation for drug/food interactions	30 min
99204	level 4	comprehensive	moderate complexity	complex medication regimen evaluation with multiple issues to address	45 min
99205	level 5	high complexity	moderate complexity	complex medication regimen evaluation with multiple issues to address and complete home blood glucose monitoring teaching	60 min

Source: Pihl-Leggett SH. Documentation and Billing for Pharmacist Care of Diabetes. Alexandria, Va: National Institute for Pharmacist Care Outcomes; 2001.

Interacting with Third-Party Payers

The basis for getting paid by Medicaid, TPAs, and PBMs is the claim for a prescription for a specific beneficiary. While in the past pharmacies have filed claims on paper or on computer magnetic tape or disks, today most interact with the claims processor in real time by direct Internet communication or modem-to-modem connection. This is called a *point-of-service system*, described in Table 11-2.

If all information has been entered correctly and verified by the claims processor, the pharmacy will then be paid for the prescription (through a process known as claims adjudication). Payment is usually made by electronic transfer into the pharmacy's designated bank account on a daily, weekly, or other periodic basis.

When there is a problem, you or the pharmacist may need to call the TPA or PBM for assistance. This is a frustrating part of daily life in the community pharmacy, as you may stay on hold for several minutes listening to the same messages or music while waiting for a person to talk with. But once you're talking with a person, be courteous, as you both have the same goal in mind: determining if this patient is eligible for this prescription at this time. The sooner you convey the nature of the problem and the faster the other person can assess the information, the sooner you both can be off the phone and on to your next tasks.

Billing for Pharmaceutical Care Services

If your pharmacist is involved in pharmaceutical care services, you will no doubt also need to be familiar with billing for these clinical activities. This type of billing involves detailing the services that have been provided, along with any laboratory tests performed in the pharmacy. While the cost of medications is usually not billed with pharmaceutical care, it might be included for services such as influenza vaccination.

Getting paid for pharmaceutical care services has been relatively rare in the past but is now increasingly common. For billing for clinical services, you need to be familiar with the following terms and forms:

Reimbursement for prescriptions is often handled through an intermediary company, such as PCS Health Systems or Medco. These companies, known as pharmacy benefits managers, or PBMs, are very important parts of the current payment system in community pharmacy.

FIGURE 11-1

Form 1500 of the Centers for Medicare & Medicaid Services.

PLEASE
DO NOT
STAPLE
IN THIS
AREA

| | PICA | | | | | | | **HEALTH INSURANCE CLAIM FORM** | | PICA |

HEALTH INSURANCE CLAIM FORM

1. MEDICARE   MEDICAID   CHAMPUS   CHAMPVA   GROUP HEALTH PLAN   FECA BLK LUNG   OTHER   1a. INSURED'S I.D. NUMBER   (FOR PROGRAM IN ITEM 1)

(Medicare #)   (Medicaid #)   (Sponsor's SSN)   (VA File #)   (SSN or ID)   (SSN)   (ID)

2. PATIENT'S NAME (Last Name, First Name, Middle Initial)

3. PATIENT'S BIRTH DATE   MM   DD   YY   SEX   M ☐   F ☐

4. INSURED'S NAME (Last Name, First Name, Middle Initial)

2nd FOLD

5. PATIENT'S ADDRESS (No., Street)

6. PATIENT RELATIONSHIP TO INSURED   Self ☐   Spouse ☐   Child ☐   Other ☐

7. INSURED'S ADDRESS (No., Street)

CITY   STATE   8. PATIENT STATUS   Single ☐   Married ☐   Other ☐

CITY   STATE

ZIP CODE   TELEPHONE (Include Area Code) ( )   Employed ☐   Full-Time Student ☐   Part-Time Student ☐

ZIP CODE   TELEPHONE (INCLUDE AREA CODE) ( )

9. OTHER INSURED'S NAME (Last Name, First Name, Middle Initial)

10. IS PATIENT'S CONDITION RELATED TO:

11. INSURED'S POLICY GROUP OR FECA NUMBER

a. OTHER INSURED'S POLICY OR GROUP NUMBER

a. EMPLOYMENT? (CURRENT OR PREVIOUS)   YES ☐   NO ☐

a. INSURED'S DATE OF BIRTH   MM   DD   YY   SEX   M ☐   F ☐

b. OTHER INSURED'S DATE OF BIRTH   MM   DD   YY   SEX   M ☐   F ☐

b. AUTO ACCIDENT?   PLACE (State)   YES ☐   NO ☐

b. EMPLOYER'S NAME OR SCHOOL NAME

c. EMPLOYER'S NAME OR SCHOOL NAME

c. OTHER ACCIDENT?   YES ☐   NO ☐

c. INSURANCE PLAN NAME OR PROGRAM NAME

d. INSURANCE PLAN NAME OR PROGRAM NAME

10d. RESERVED FOR LOCAL USE

d. IS THERE ANOTHER HEALTH BENEFIT PLAN?   YES ☐   NO ☐   *If yes*, return to and complete item 9 a-d.

READ BACK OF FORM BEFORE COMPLETING & SIGNING THIS FORM.

12. PATIENT'S OR AUTHORIZED PERSON'S SIGNATURE I authorize the release of any medical or other information necessary to process this claim. I also request payment of government benefits either to myself or to the party who accepts assignment below.

SIGNED _____   DATE _____

13. INSURED'S OR AUTHORIZED PERSON'S SIGNATURE I authorize payment of medical benefits to the undersigned physician or supplier for services described below.

SIGNED _____

1st FOLD

14. DATE OF CURRENT: MM   DD   YY   ILLNESS (First symptom) OR INJURY (Accident) OR PREGNANCY(LMP)

15. IF PATIENT HAS HAD SAME OR SIMILAR ILLNESS. GIVE FIRST DATE   MM   DD   YY

16. DATES PATIENT UNABLE TO WORK IN CURRENT OCCUPATION   MM   DD   YY   FROM   TO   MM   DD   YY

17. NAME OF REFERRING PHYSICIAN OR OTHER SOURCE

17a. I.D. NUMBER OF REFERRING PHYSICIAN

18. HOSPITALIZATION DATES RELATED TO CURRENT SERVICES   MM   DD   YY   FROM   TO   MM   DD   YY

19. RESERVED FOR LOCAL USE

20. OUTSIDE LAB? $ CHARGES   YES ☐   NO ☐

21. DIAGNOSIS OR NATURE OF ILLNESS OR INJURY. (RELATE ITEMS 1,2,3 OR 4 TO ITEM 24E BY LINE)

1. |___.___   3. |___.___

2. |___.___   4. |___.___

22. MEDICAID RESUBMISSION CODE   ORIGINAL REF. NO.

23. PRIOR AUTHORIZATION NUMBER

24.	A				B	C	D		E	F	G	H	I	J	K
	DATE(S) OF SERVICE				Place of Service	Type of Service	PROCEDURES, SERVICES, OR SUPPLIES (Explain Unusual Circumstances)		DIAGNOSIS CODE	$ CHARGES	DAYS OR UNITS	EPSDT Family Plan	EMG	COB	RESERVED FOR LOCAL USE
	From		To				CPT/HCPCS	MODIFIER							
	MM DD YY		MM DD YY												
1															
2															
3															
4															
5															
6															

25. FEDERAL TAX I.D. NUMBER   SSN ☐   EIN ☐

26. PATIENT'S ACCOUNT NO.

27. ACCEPT ASSIGNMENT? (For govt. claims, see back)   YES ☐   NO ☐

28. TOTAL CHARGE $

29. AMOUNT PAID $

30. BALANCE DUE $

01002

FIGURE 11-2

Pharmacist Care Claim Form, as Developed by the National Community Pharmacists Association.

Subscriber Information

Name	Phone
Address	SUBMIT TO ▶
City	State	Zip	REFERENCE #
Birthdate	Sex M F	Social Security Subscriber I.D. No.	Date of Service	HCFA-1500 attached ☐

PATIENT AUTHORIZATION
I hereby authorize release of information to health care providers, institutions, and/or payers that may pertain to my illness and/or treatment received. I certify that the information I have reported with regard to my insurance coverage is correct, and I have received the pharmacist care/service rendered.

Employer	Employer I.D.
Group No.	Plan No.

Patient Signature   Date

Patient

Name	Birthdate	Sex M F

Relationship of Patient to Subscriber ☐ Self ☐ Spouse ☐ Child ☐ Other

---

Pharmacist Care Information

I. REASON FOR SERVICE

ADMINISTRATIVE
____ Call Help Desk	CH
____ Drug Not Available	NA
____ Lock-In Recipient	LK
____ Missiing Informatin/Clarification	MS
____ New Patient Processing	NP
____ Non-Covered Drug Purchase	NC
____ Non-Formulary Drug	NF
____ Payer/Processor Question	TP
____ Prescription Authentication	AN
____ Product Selection Opportunity	PS

DOSING/LIMITS
____ Excessive Duration	MX
____ Excessive Quantity	EX
____ High Dose	HD
____ Insufficient Duration	MN
____ Insufficient Quantity	NS
____ Low Dose	LD
____ Overuse	ER
____ Suboptimal Compliance	SC
____ Suboptimal Dosage Form	SF
____ Suboptimal Regimen	SR
____ Underuse	LR

DRUG CONFLICT
____ Additive Toxcity	AT
____ Drug-Age Precaution	PA
____ Drug-Allergy	DA
____ Drug-Disease (Reported)	MC
____ Drug-Disease (Inferred)	DC
____ Drug-Drug Interactions	DD
____ Drug-Gender	SX
____ Drug Incompatibility	DI

____ Drug-Pregnancy	PG
____ Iatrogenic Condition	IC
____ Ingredient Duplication	ID
____ Lactation/Nursing Interaction	NR
____ Prior Adverse Drug Reaction	PR
____ Therapeutic Duplication	TD

DISEASE MANAGEMENT
____ Additional Drug Needed	AD
____ Adverse Drug Reaction	AR
____ Apparent Drug Misuse	DM
____ Chronic Disease Management	CD
____ Health Provider Referral	RF
____ Laboratory Test Needed	TN
____ New Disease/Diagnosis	ND
____ Patient Complaint/Symptom	CS
____ Patient Education/Instruction	ED
____ Patient Question/Concern	PC
____ Plan Protocol	PP
____ Preventive Health Care	PH
____ Prescriber Consultation	PN
____ Suboptimal Drug/Indication	SD
____ Suspected Environmental Risk	RE
____ Unnecessary Drug	NN

PRECAUTIONARY
____ Alcohol Precaution	OH
____ Drug-Food Interaction	DF
____ Drug Lab-Conflict	DI
____ Side Effect	SE
____ Tobacco Use Precaution	DS
____ Other (specify below)	97

II. PROFESSIONAL SERVICE

ADMINISTRATIVE
____ Formulary Enforcement	FE
____ Generic Product Selection	GP
____ Literature Search/Review	SW
____ Patient Medication History	PH
____ Payer/Processor Consulted	TC
____ Therapeutic Product Interchange	TH

PATIENT CARE
____ Coordination Of Care	CC
____ Dosing Evaluation/Determination	DE
____ Medication Administration	MA
____ Medication Review	MR
____ Patient Assessment	AS
____ Patient Consulted	PØ
____ Patient Education/Instruction	PE
____ Patient Monitoring	PM
____ Perform Laboratory Test	PT
____ Pharmacist Consulted Other Source	RØ
____ Prescriber Consulted	MØ
____ Recommended Laboratory Test	RT
____ Self-Care Consultation	SC
____ Other (specify below)	98

III. RESULT OF SERVICE

DISPENSED
____ Brand for Generic Change	1H
____ Filled As Is False Positive	1B
____ Filled Prescription As Is	1B
____ Filled With Different Directions	1D
____ Filled With Different Dosage Form	1K
____ Filled With Different Dose	1C
____ Filled With Different Drug	1E
____ Filled With Different Quantity	1F
____ Filled With Prescriber Approval	1G
____ Rx-to-OTC Change	1J

NOT DISPENSED
____ Not Filled, Directions Clarified	2B
____ Prescription Not Filled	2A

PATIENT CARE
____ Compliance Aid Provided	2B
____ Discontinued Drug	3C
____ Drug Therapy Unchanged	3G
____ Follow-Up Report	3H
____ Instructions Understood	3K
____ Medication Administered	3N
____ Patient Referral	3J
____ Recommendation Accepted	3A
____ Recommendation Not Accepted	3B
____ Regimen Changed	3D
____ Therapy Changed	3F
____ Therapy Changed	3F
____ Cost Increase Acknowledged	
____ Other (specify below)	99

IV. LEVEL OF SERVICE

Level 1 (Lowest) = 11	Level 4 = 14	
Level 2 = 12	Level 5 (Highest) = 15	
Level 3 = 13		

V. DRUGS INVOLVED (IF APPLICABLE)

NDC: [   ]   NDC: [   ]

VI. BILLING CODE/PROFESSIONAL FEE   FEE

DISCUSSION

I am certified to provide pharmacist care for:	☐ Anticoagulation	☐ Immunizations	☐ Lipid Disorders	☐ Osteoporosis	☐ Other
	☐ Arthritis	☐ Infectious diseases	☐ Mental Health	☐ Ostomy/incontinence/wounds	
	☐ Asthma/Resp. Condition	☐ Hormone Replacement Therapy	☐ Nutrition/wellness	☐ Pain Management	
	☐ Diabetes	☐ Hypertension	☐ Orthotics/prosthetics	☐ Reproductive Health	

Pharmacy Imprint

NAME	TELEPHONE
ADDRESS	

I hereby certify that the pharmacist care rendered as indicated has been completed and the fee submitted is the actual fee I have charged and intend to collect for this service.

Signature of Pharmacist ▶

NCPCP/NABP NO.	SSN/TIN
Date	Pharmacist ID

WHITE - PAYER   YELLOW - PATIENT   PINK - PHARMACY/OTHER

TABLE 11-4

CPT Codes Used Most Frequently by Pharmacists for Established Patients

CODE	LEVEL	HISTORY	DECISION	EXAMPLES	TIME
99211	level 1	minimal	straightforward	review basics of oral agent/insulin with patient who has been on agent in past	5 min
99212	level 2	problem-focused	straightforward	complete education provided for the patient receiving oral agent/insulin for the first time	10 min
99213	level 3	expanded problem-focused	low complexity	complete education of oral agent/insulin and evaluation for drug/food interactions	15 min
99214	level 4	detailed	moderate complexity	complex medication regimen evaluation with multiple issues to address	25 min
99215	level 5	comprehensive	high complexity	complex medication regimen evaluation with multiple issues to address and complete home blood glucose monitoring teaching	40 min

Source: Pihl-Leggett SH. Documentation and Billing for Pharmacist Care of Diabetes. Alexandria, Va: National Institute for Pharmacist Care Outcomes; 2001.

Getting paid for pharmaceutical care services has been relatively rare in the past but is now increasingly common.

- **CPT Codes** — Common Procedural Terminology (CPT) codes are used to describe clinical interactions with patients. These codes vary according to (1) whether the patient is a new or an established patient, (2) the complexity of the clinical situation, and (3) the amount of time the pharmacist spends with the patient. The 10 CPT codes that have been used by pharmacists are shown in Tables 11-3 and 11-4. A coalition of pharmacy organizations, the Pharmacist Services Technical Advisory Coalition (www.pstac.org), is seeking recognition of Category I (permanent) CPT codes that can be used for billing medication therapy management services. Toward that end, the Category III (temporary) CPT codes for medication therapy management services shown in Table 11-5 were established in 2005. The coalition was presenting evidence supporting making these codes permanent when this book was finalized in early 2007.

- **ICD-9 Codes** — The International Classification of Diseases, 9th Revision, Clinical Modification is a set of standard numbers used for designating patients' diseases. Because the physician makes the diagnosis of patients' conditions, the pharmacist must simply obtain the correct ICD-9 code from the physician to use on the reimbursement forms. However, an error in entering this code will cause rejection of the claim.

- **HCPCS Codes** — The Healthcare Common Procedure Coding System (HCPCS) codes are used for billing for medical devices (such as walkers, wheelchairs, syringes, and medication administration sets). These consist of a letter and four numbers. Codes beginning with letters A–R and T–V describe supplies and medications and are the same throughout the United States. Codes that start with the letters S or W–Z are established by local Medicare carriers for claims for physician services, such as laboratory tests or surgical procedures.

- **CMS 1500 Form** — The CMS 1500 Form, shown in Figure 11-1, is a commonly used form for billing pharmaceutical care services. This form is the same one used by many physicians for billing office visits. Pharmacists use the various boxes on the form to convey to the third-party administrator or payer the kinds of services that were provided to the patient.
- **Pharmacist Care Claim Form** — Shown in Figure 11-2, the Pharmacist Care Claim Form (PCCF) was developed by the National Community Pharmacists Association to provide pharmacists with a more specific way of billing for their clinical services. While many payers still do not recognize the PCCF, pharmacists often file it with the CMS 1500 because it provides an important increased level of detail that can convince payers of the utility of pharmacists' services.

TABLE 11-5

Category III MTM CPT Codes Approved in 2005

0115T	Medication therapy management service(s) provided by a pharmacist, individual, face-to-face with patient, initial 15 minutes, with assessment, and intervention if provided; initial encounter
0116T	Subsequent encounter
+0117T	Each additional 15 minutes (list separately in addition to code for primary service; use 0117T in conjunction with 0115T, 0116T)

Source: Pharmacist Services Technical Advisory Coalition and Current Procedural Terminology—CPT 2007. 4th ed. Chicago, Ill.: American Medical Association; 2007.

Reimbursement is the important last step in the process of dispensing prescriptions.

Conclusion

Reimbursement is the important last step in the process of dispensing prescriptions. Without adequate flow of cash from Medicare Part D, Medicaid, and other third-party payers, few pharmacies would survive in today's environment.

As this chapter closes out Part II, we now turn our attention to some of the processes and systems that help keep most pharmacies functioning smoothly. Maintenance of adequate inventory is the first such system we will explore as we begin Part III and Chapter 12.

More Information

If you are preparing for the Pharmacy Technician Certification Examination and feel that you need more information about the topics discussed in this chapter, consider studying these sources of additional information:

- Desselle SP, Zgarrick DP. *Pharmacy Management: Essentials for All Practice Settings.* New York: McGraw-Hill; 2005.
- News stories about Medicare and Medicaid reimbursement posted in 2007 or later on APhA's www.pharmacist.com Web site.
- Touchette DR, Burns AL, Bough MA, Blackburn JC. Survey of medication therapy management programs under Medicare Part D. *J Am Pharm Assoc.* 2006;46:683–91.
- Boyd ST, Boyd LC, Zillich AJ. Medication therapy management survey of the prescription drug plans. *J Am Pharm Assoc.* 2006;46:692–9.

References

Current Procedural Terminology—CPT 2007. 4th ed. Chicago, Ill.: American Medical Association; 2007.

American Medical Association. *International Classification of Diseases. 9th revision, clinical modification*. Chicago, IL: American Medical Association; 1998.

National Institute for Pharmacist Care Outcomes. *NIPCO-Accredited Diabetes Care Program*. Alexandria, VA: National Institute for Pharmacist Care Outcomes; 1998.

Schafermeyer KW. Basics of managed care claims processing: from claims payment to outcomes management. *J Managed Care Pharm*. 1995;1:200–5.

Thomas N, Larson L. Pharmacy reimbursement in managed care. In: Navarro R, Wertheimer A, eds. *Managing the Pharmacy Benefit*. Warren, NJ: Emron, Inc.; 1996:47–63.

PART III

Maintaining Medication and Inventory Control Systems

CHAPTER TWELVE

Inventory Control and Management

In many pharmacies, technicians specialize in assisting with the purchase of pharmaceuticals and other needed products. This chapter provides background for technicians who aspire to a position in this area, as well as basic information that all pharmacy technicians need to know.

As a worker whose job involves handling your pharmacy's inventory, you can help make the best use of this investment.

Introduction

The job of any manager in the business sector is to create an environment in which the financial and human resources of the firm are used to generate a profit. Even in a small pharmacy, considerable financial resources are invested in the goods for sale. With drug prices being as high as they are, several hundred thousand dollars are tied up in the inventory, equipment, and fixtures of each pharmacy.

As a worker whose job involves handling your pharmacy's inventory, you can help make the best use of this investment. In addition, in hospital pharmacies and larger community stores, some technicians specialize in purchasing; they spend the majority of their time checking inventory levels, placing orders, and following up on items not received. Let's look at inventory management and the role you will play in it.

Managing Inventory

Think of a newspaper rack in front of your neighborhood coffee shop. During the night, the newspaper carrier puts 10 morning newspapers into the rack. When that carrier returns the next day, what is the ideal number of newspapers that should be remaining?

If sales are to be maximized, then obviously the carrier would like to see an empty rack—all the newspapers were sold. However, the carrier would then wonder how many sales had been lost because the rack was empty. In this situation, it is better for the carrier to find one newspaper remaining in the rack, because that means that as many newspapers as possible were sold without losing any sales.

Inventory management in the pharmacy is similar to this newspaper analogy. You never want to run out of any drug, but you want to keep as little as possible on hand so that *inventory costs* are minimized. Inventory costs are discussed in Table 12-1.

To understand some approaches to managing pharmacy inventory, you must first be familiar with where pharmacies obtain the products they sell. Here are the major sources of pharmaceutical products:

The drug wholesaler is a "middle man" in the pharmaceutical supply chain.

- **Manufacturer** — The manufacturer is the company or entity that is manufacturing, distributing, and marketing the drug product and may sell it directly to the pharmacy. The pharmacy can often get lower prices when it purchases products directly from the manufacturer, but it also has to order certain minimum quantities.
- **Wholesaler** — The drug wholesaler is a "middle man" in the pharmaceutical supply chain. Wholesalers stock many thousands of items that are generally found in pharmacies, from health and beauty aids to nonprescription agents to the most expensive prescription drugs. As wholesalers have become heavily computerized,

---

TABLE 12-1

Inventory Costs

What are inventory costs? They include:

- The *cost of the space* where inventory is stored includes rent or mortgage payments, electricity and other utilities, and pharmacy shelving used for product displays or storage. The greater the inventory is, the higher the costs.
- The *cost of the drug products* can be several hundred dollars for one small container.

- The *value of the money* tied up in inventory might include finance charges if the inventory was purchased on credit or with borrowed money. It also includes the revenue that could have been generated if the money had been put in a savings account or invested in stocks or bonds.

they have helped pharmacies to improve their business, financial, and sales analyses based on purchasing patterns. Wholesalers have helped pharmacies take advantage of bar-coding technology in reordering products (see Figure 12-1), and they are now becoming linked in real time to pharmacy computer systems so that reordering of items sold can happen on a daily or other periodic basis.

- **Purchasing group** — Both hospital and community pharmacies have banded together to increase their purchasing power. By all committing to the use of certain common items—often intravenous fluids and administration sets but perhaps also specific drugs in commonly used therapeutic categories— members of these purchasing groups can negotiate very favorable prices with manufacturers, wholesalers, or both.

- **Prime vendor** — Pharmacies have also entered into contracts with wholesalers under which the wholesaler is promised a large percentage of the business from that pharmacy. These wholesalers, referred to as prime vendors for that pharmacy, in return give special pricing and assistance to the pharmacy in managing inventory levels and costs.

- **Other pharmacies** — When one pharmacy runs out of an item or needs a product they do not usually stock, the staff often borrows from another pharmacy. Ask your pharmacist what other pharmacies in your area you generally contact for this purpose.

In placing orders, many pharmacies use a calculated economic order quantity (EOQ), as follows:

$$EOQ = \sqrt{\frac{2LM}{W}}$$

L = annual purchases of the item in dollars
M = dollar cost of reordering or issuing a purchase order
W = cost of capital or carrying inventory (interest rate on borrowed funds)

As illustrated in Figure 12-2, the use of the EOQ system creates three critical numbers. First, the EOQ is the ideal amount of inventory that should be ordered so that the costs of carrying the inventory and the costs of reordering and stocking the inventory are minimized. Next, a reorder level must be determined, based on how fast the product is selling and how long it takes to get a new order in. Finally, an emergency level is designated so that special actions (for example, telephone calls, ordering from a different source, borrowing) can be taken if the inventory gets too low before the order comes in.

As computerization has increased managers' ability to track inventory levels and overnight delivery services have become available, many managers have adopted a "just-in-time" inventory system. As the name suggests, this system is designed to have inventory arrive just as the previous supply is exhausted. For items whose usage and delivery are predictable, this system helps to minimize pharmacy inventory costs and stocking levels.

FIGURE 12-1

Bar-coding.

Bar-coding of pharmaceutical products helps with inventory control and the ordering process. Bar codes are also increasingly used during the dispensing process to make sure the product matches the prescription order; in hospitals, nurses also use bar codes on patients' wristbands to make sure the drug, the patient, the route of administration, and the time of administration are all correct.

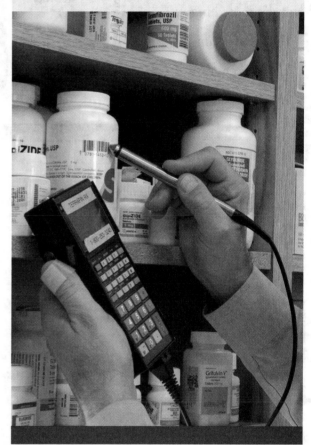

Both hospital and community pharmacies have banded together to increase their purchasing power.

The process of placing orders for pharmaceuticals has become very streamlined as computer and bar code technology has eliminated many time-consuming manual chores.

FIGURE 12-2

Application of the Economic Order Quantity in Inventory Management.

Inventory (No. Units)

Economic Order Quantity

Reorder point

Emergency action point

Time

FIGURE 12-3

Orders to pharmacy wholesalers can be placed using automated or manual online systems.

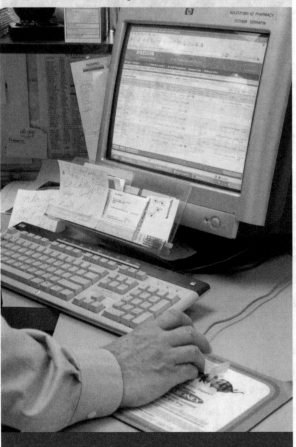

Placing Orders

The process of placing orders for pharmaceuticals has become very streamlined as computer and bar code technology has eliminated many time-consuming manual chores. Now, rather than reading from a handwritten list of items, the pharmacist or technician can simply upload an order from the computer or, using handheld devices, walk around the store scanning bar codes from labels attached to shelving. Or, as mentioned above, they may not need to do anything—the pharmacy computer may have automatically reordered from the wholesaler everything sold each day (see Figure 12-3).

Even though the process is becoming increasingly simplified, that does not mean it is any less critical. Whatever role you are asked to play in ordering merchandise, you should approach the task with the same accuracy and care that you use in filling patients' prescriptions. Make sure you understand what the pharmacist or owner expects, what their views are on inventory management, and how often orders are normally placed.

In addition to computerized systems, pharmacies may still have some vestige of a manual "want book" for making notes about special items that customers have asked for or unusual products that are needed. The want book, once the major method of recording needed merchandise, is generally a spiral-bound notebook that all employees use for making notes of orders to be placed. The person who places orders will go through the list, reconcile the items with those already ordered electronically or automatically, and add needed products to the order.

Receiving Orders

When orders arrive from either the manufacturer or the wholesaler, they should be accompanied by either an invoice or a packing slip that lists what the pharmacy is being charged for. As you remove the items from the box and place them into inventory, it is critical that you check them against this list; otherwise, the pharmacy may not receive everything it will be asked to pay for.

Also be sure to follow any internal pharmacy procedures concerning the receipt of inventory. For instance, you may need to confirm receipt of the order in the pharmacy computer system, either through manual entry or by bar-coding the incoming items. Unless you let the computer know that the order has been received, it will reflect an incorrect inventory level and may keep trying to order more product even though an adequate amount is on hand.

If your order contains controlled substances, you will need to follow special procedures to check these in. As mentioned in Chapter 3, DEA order form 222, supplied in triplicate, is used for ordering Schedule II controlled substances. Copy 3 is filed at the pharmacy. When the order is received, copy 3 of the DEA form 222 is pulled from the pharmacy files. The person processing the order records on copy 3 the date and amount of drug product received. Copy 3 is then refiled and kept for 2 years.

Conclusion

Inventory management is a very important part of pharmacy practice, and technicians are playing key roles in managing this valuable asset of the pharmacy business. However, ordering, receiving, and dispensing this inventory is only part of the story. Let's look at Chapter 13 to learn more about which drug products are used, how they are stored, and what happens when they must be returned to the manufacturer or when they are stolen.

For More Information

If you are preparing for the Pharmacy Technician Certification Examination and feel that you need more information about the topics discussed in this chapter, consider studying these sources of additional information:

- Peterson AM. Principles of inventory management. In: *Managing Pharmacy Practice: Principles, Strategies, and Systems*. Boca Raton, Fla.: CRC Press; 2004.
- Wilkin NE. General operations management. In: Desselle SP, Zgarrick DP. *Pharmacy Management: Essentials for All Practice Settings*. New York: McGraw-Hill; 2005:95–108.

Whatever role you are asked to play in ordering merchandise, you should approach the task with the same accuracy and care that you use in filling patients' prescriptions.

Be sure to follow any internal pharmacy procedures concerning the receipt of inventory.

References

Peterson AM. Principles of inventory management. In: *Managing Pharmacy Practice: Principles, Strategies, and Systems.* Boca Raton, Fla.: CRC Press; 2004.

Tootelian DH, Gaedeke RM. Operations management and computerizing the pharmacy. In: *Essentials of Pharmacy Management.* St. Louis, MO: Mosby–Year Book; 1993:383–6.

Wilkin NE. General operations management. In: Desselle SP, Zgarrick DP. *Pharmacy Management: Essentials for All Practice Settings.* New York: McGraw-Hill; 2005:95–108.

CHAPTER THIRTEEN

Special Considerations: Drug Formularies, Storage, Recalls, and Theft and Diversion

Chapter 13 describes the interplay between the pharmaceutical industry, regulatory agencies, managed care organizations, third-party payers, and the pharmacy. In covering drug formularies, medication-storage requirements, product recalls, and the need to protect against theft or diversion of controlled substances, this chapter places pharmacy practice into a larger perspective.

Introduction

As noted in the last chapter, pharmacy inventory is critical to commercial success. Without access to the right drug product at the time that a patient needs it, the value a pharmacist can provide is considerably diminished.

However, no pharmacy can keep every prescription and nonprescription drug product in stock. With several thousand such products on the US market, all pharmacies must be selective. Not only are the costs of storage and display prohibitive, unneeded products simply drive up the cost of inventory and increase the potential for theft or damage without a related increase in sales and profits. In addition, pharmaceutical products can only be sold while they are in date; after the expiration date printed on each container, the product must be returned to the manufacturer or discarded. Other things can also go wrong: The manufacturer may recall the product for many different reasons, or the product may be shoplifted by a patient or stolen by an employee of the pharmacy.

In this chapter, we consider several advanced aspects of inventory management, including the following:

- Management of the drug formulary
- Proper storage of pharmaceuticals
- Manufacturer or FDA recall of pharmaceuticals
- Diversion and theft of drug products

Drug Formularies and Policies

In hospital, managed care, and some long-term care systems and in the Medicare Part D program, physicians and financial managers working in concert with pharmacists have established lists of preferred drug products. The lists, called *formularies*, specify which medications or drug products are to be used for patients in the system. In institutions and many managed care organizations, formulary decisions are made by a committee of the medical (physician) staff, the *pharmacy and therapeutics committee*. The committee includes a representative of the medical staff and generally a pharmacist and a nurse.

Medications and products are selected for inclusion on the formulary by using four criteria to compare them with other available products, as discussed in Table 13-1.

By shifting pharmaceutical use toward formulary agents, the health system enjoys several benefits. First, in many cases, patients are treated with more effective and/or safer medications. They get well faster, are better protected against disease, and have fewer side effects and detrimental drug interactions. The health system is able to eliminate other medications and drug products from its inventory, saving on the inventory and related costs. Second, the system also purchases larger quantities of the formulary agents, which may enable it to receive larger discounts from the manufacturer or wholesaler. Third, if the health system is dominant enough in a given geographic area, it may be able to negotiate even larger discounts based on its ability to guarantee certain usage levels of the product to the manufacturer.

Occasionally a health system will add a drug to its formulary but place it in a restricted category. Usually this is done because the drug has serious side effects, is difficult to use properly, or is very expensive. Only certain types of physician specialists are allowed to prescribe the restricted drug, or general practitioner

---

TABLE 13-1

Criteria for Inclusion on the Formulary

Medications and products are selected for inclusion on the formulary by using these four criteria:

- Better effectiveness against the disease in question
- Fewer side effects
- Better pharmacokinetic profiles, including fewer drug interactions with food or other drugs, laboratory tests, or fewer number of daily doses
- Lower costs

physicians (including family medicine physicians and pediatricians) are required to get permission from physician specialists before they prescribe it.

Another common formulary policy involves automatic stop orders. In this case, physicians instruct the pharmacy to automatically stop therapy with certain medications unless the prescribing physician reorders them or asks for the agents to be continued. This is most commonly done with antibiotics, which need to be reassessed a few days after they are begun when certain laboratory tests become available.

While the utility and effectiveness of drug formularies is not universally supported, they have definitely proven useful for limiting pharmacy inventories and directing physician prescribers toward preferred agents. You are sure to see formularies used in hospital and large health systems, and community pharmacies routinely must deal with formularies of various managed care plans and third-party payers.

Storage of Pharmaceutical Products

Medications—which are really just chemicals that affect the human body in some beneficial way—are often sensitive to changes in temperature, light, humidity, or other environmental factors. Because of their delicate nature, medications must be stored under specified conditions so that they do not degrade—that is, change into chemicals that have no effect or are harmful when used on or in the body.

Storage conditions are defined when a drug is first approved for marketing in the United States. The FDA approves the storage conditions for drug products based on data and information supplied by the manufacturer. The official categories for drug storage are in Table 4-3.

In addition, the United States Pharmacopeial Convention (USP) issues monographs that define how drugs should be stored and what variance is allowed in their stated contents. Some drugs are not dangerous after they degrade, or most people are not very sensitive to variations in the dose of that drug. Such drugs can still be used even if the amount of drug remaining has fallen as low as 85% or 90% of the amount stated on the label. But other drugs degrade to more detrimental compounds, or their dosages need to be precise to be effective and not cause side effects when people take them. For those products, USP might require that the product not degrade beyond 95% of labeled amounts.

The manufacturer combines the FDA and USP considerations about its drug to calculate an expiration date for the product based on studies that show how quickly the drug degrades under approved storage conditions. Use of the drug product beyond this date is not allowed under federal and state laws in the United States.

Many pharmaceutical manufacturers use every-6-month dating, meaning that expiration dates are set in June and December of each year. For these products, you will need to go through the inventory of the pharmacy only twice a year looking for expired drugs. However, other companies assign expiration dates based on the actual month a product is expected to drop below the allowable limit, and these must be removed monthly.

Most pharmacies now have expiration dates in their computer systems, so you may be able to work from an expired drugs list in pulling old products. Without this list, removal of expired drug products can be a tiring and never-ending chore.

Most manufacturers have policies and procedures about (1) whether the pharmacy can get credit for the expired drug products and (2) how much credit is allowed and what the pharmacy must do to get the credit (for example, give the expired drugs to a sales representative or destroy the expired drugs and sign a statement attesting to the type and quantity). If the expired products are controlled substances as scheduled by the Drug Enforcement Administration, then other rules and regulations apply to the drugs. Be sure to work with

Medications must be stored under specified conditions so that they do not degrade—that is, change into chemicals that have no effect or are harmful when used on or in the body.

The presence of controlled substances— narcotics, amphetamines, sleeping pills, and sometimes cocaine—makes pharmacies a target for addicts looking for their preferred substance of abuse or criminals who want to sell the drugs on illicit markets.

your pharmacist in handling expired drug products so that the pharmacy can recoup these costs and so that no laws are broken.

Pharmacy computer systems generally put a 1-year expiration date on prescription labels; the patient is instructed to throw the medication away after 1 year regardless of the original manufacturer's date. Several factors should be remembered about this type of dating:

- The reason for the arbitrary 1-year date is that many consumers do not store the drug product under FDA-defined conditions. For instance, many people keep their medications in either the kitchen or the bathroom. The kitchen is generally the hottest room in the house, so medications stored there will be subjected to excessive heat, especially if the family's house is not air-conditioned. The bathroom is the most humid room in most homes, and humidity is the most important factor in degradation for many drugs. Thus, even if the manufacturer's original expiration date is several years away, a 1-year expiration date is used for prescriptions at the time of dispensing.

- In areas with especially hot or humid climates, you should advise patients to keep their prescription medications in areas where the temperature and humidity are controlled. In particular, advise patients not to expose prescription drugs to excessive heat by leaving them in hot automobiles on warm days.

- If you are dispensing a prescription drug product with less than 1 year remaining in the company's expiration date, then you must place that date on the patient's prescription label instead of the standard 1-year date.

USP issues standards that govern the conditions under which medications should be stored as they move through distribution channels, from manufacturer to wholesaler to pharmacy to patient. As was discussed in the Medication Storage section of Chapter 8, these requirements sometimes mean that products must be placed on ice or otherwise refrigerated during shipment. In addition, pharmaceutical sales representatives who store drug samples in their cars must take care during periods of hot or cold weather to ensure the integrity of those medications.

Recalls of Drug Products

Sometimes, despite FDA's and manufacturers' best efforts, drug products must be recalled from the market. While these recalls are usually termed "voluntary" (meaning that the company has recalled the product on its own), almost all are actually negotiated with FDA beforehand.

FDA places recalls into three categories based on the seriousness of the problem and the relative risk to public health in general. Refer to Chapter 3 for a description of the three categories.

As with expired medications, you must follow specific instructions from

FIGURE 13-1

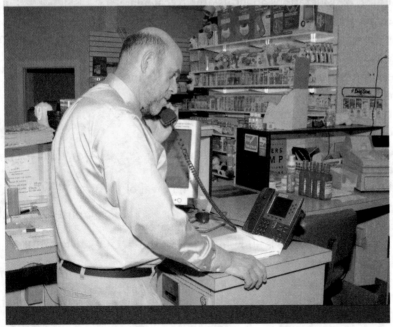

When prescription or other medications are recalled, pharmacies need to notify patients of the need to stop taking the drugs and the procedure for returning unused product for credit.

the manufacturer so that the pharmacy can get its money back for recalled products. In addition, pharmacies must contact patients whose prescriptions were dispensed using recalled drug products (or, when the pharmacy can track this, nonprescription drug products that consumers have purchased over the counter). Follow the policies and procedures in your pharmacy for how these notifications are to be handled (for example, mail, phone, fax, or e-mail), considering the relative seriousness of the recall (Figure 13-1).

Theft and Diversion of Drugs

All pharmacies must have precautions in place to guard against the theft of money or drugs through burglary, robbery, or shoplifting. But an equally important concern is internal theft of money and diversion of medications by employees of the pharmacy or other personnel in institutions such as hospitals and nursing homes.

As a technician, you need to be familiar with the actions expected of you if a crime is taking place. You also need to realize how dangerous some medicines are and how easily employees can become addicted to narcotics or become involved in diverting drugs to illegal markets for personal profit.

The presence of controlled substances—narcotics, amphetamines, sleeping pills, and sometimes cocaine—makes pharmacies a target for addicts looking for their preferred substance of abuse or criminals who want to sell the drugs on illicit markets. As with most retail outlets, community pharmacies are sometimes the targets of criminals looking to steal money or shoplift merchandise. Hospital pharmacies have even been targeted for robberies and burglaries because of the quantities and types of controlled substances stored there. Some pharmacies intersperse Schedule III, IV, and V controlled substances in the general medication storage areas, but Schedule II drugs are kept in locked cabinets (see Figure 13-2), vaults, or safes.

Because of these dangers, pharmacies must have action plans in place for employees to follow if they know or believe that a crime is in progress. You should talk with the management of your pharmacy if you have not been told what to do in the event of robbery, burglary, or shoplifting. If you are not comfortable with the action being requested, you should talk with your supervisor about your feelings. Potential situations and possible measures you may be asked to take are discussed in Table 13-2.

While often not given the same emphasis as external thefts, internal theft of money, merchandise, and medications is an equally serious concern for the pharmacy owner and manager. Pharmacy managers may ask you to become bonded (a type of insurance) if your job involves handling money. Most pharmacies take any problems with missing cash seriously. Be careful when handling money, and be sure you understand the pharmacy's policies and procedures about how cash should be handled. Even if you become one of the most trusted employees in the pharmacy, you must still be watched.

FIGURE 13-2

Cabinets such as this one are used in some pharmacies for storage of controlled substances.

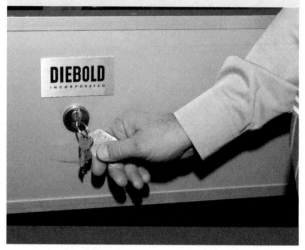

All pharmacies must have precautions in place to guard against the theft of money or drugs through burglary, robbery, or shoplifting.

FIGURE 13-3

Mirrors are used in pharmacies so that employees can watch for shoplifters.

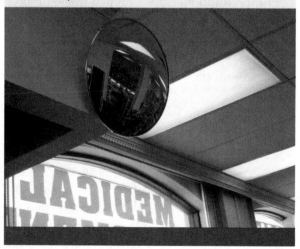

TABLE 13-2

Robbery, Burglary, and Shoplifting

In the case of a robbery, burglary, or shoplifting incident at your pharmacy, you may be instructed to consider the following:

- **Robbery:** Robbery usually involves threats by criminals brandishing firearms or other weapons. It is usually the most dangerous situation that can occur in a pharmacy. Especially when the perpetrator is an addict seeking drugs, pharmacy personnel are facing a desperate person who may harm or kill anyone who does not comply with his or her demands. The most common recommendation is to give the robber whatever is requested. Many pharmacies have buttons located near cash registers and in the prescription department that will alert the police to the crime in progress. If one of these can be discreetly activated, it will get help on the way.

- **Burglary:** Burglaries occur when the pharmacy is closed. Thus, the situation you might encounter is finding the results of a burglary when you come to work to open the pharmacy. Another common scenario could occur when the pharmacy's security system is activated; if you are a contact person for the pharmacy, you might be called by the security company or the police to check the pharmacy to see if anything is wrong. For two reasons, it is best to not enter the pharmacy, or to leave if you have already entered, if

you discover a burglary: (1) the burglars might still be in the pharmacy, and (2) you don't want to change the crime scene until after the police have investigated and possibly taken fingerprints.

- **Shoplifting:** The theft of merchandise is undoubtedly the most common crime in the pharmacy. In larger community stores, several antishoplifting devices may be in use, including cameras, reflectors (see Figure 13-3), one-way mirrors, or even security officers. Your job as a pharmacy technician will not generally involve watching for shoplifters, but you should be very familiar with the policies and procedures of the pharmacy so that you will know what is expected when you encounter a shoplifting situation. Most pharmacy owners and managers take shoplifting very seriously and prosecute those involved. First of all, because most pharmacies only clear a small profit on each sale, they need to generate many dollars in sales to recoup the theft of $1 worth of merchandise. Second, failure to prosecute shoplifters sends the message that there is little risk in trying—if shoplifters are not caught, they get the merchandise; if they are caught, they just give the goods back and walk out.

Do not be insulted if your supervisor or the pharmacy owner or manager asks you questions or double-checks your activities when it comes to money.

Theft of merchandise by employees is a serious situation. It has the same effect on the pharmacy's financial performance as does shoplifting.

Likewise, theft of merchandise by employees is a serious situation. It has the same effect on the pharmacy's financial performance as does shoplifting. Owners and managers must deal with the attitude of some employees that one of the "benefits" of employment is taking items from the workplace for their own personal use. This is not true, and the consequences of bending the rules in this area can be termination from employment and even prosecution for theft.

When the items taken from the pharmacy are prescription medications, the situation becomes even more serious. Not only is theft involved, but the federal law requiring a prescription order has been violated. In hospitals and nursing homes, medications may be diverted by nurses, physicians, and other personnel (including nonprofessional staff such as housekeepers) who have access to drugs in patient-care areas. Prescriptions are required for these medications because their use needs to be monitored by a qualified prescriber, usually a physician. Do not fall into the trap of thinking you can treat yourself using prescription drugs—particularly if you have to steal them to begin with.

The most serious situation involving internal diversion of prescription medications is the theft of controlled substances (those in Schedules II, III, IV, and V, as defined in Chapter 3). These drugs are addicting, that is, people become "hooked" on them. Once addicted, people must take the drugs regularly—perhaps even several times a day—to avoid physical or psychological withdrawal symptoms. The symptoms can be severe, as in the case of the alcoholic who is shaking and vomiting or the heroin addict experiencing severe cramps, diarrhea, sweating, and insomnia (inability to sleep). Do not think that you can't become addicted—anyone can. In fact, most studies show that health professionals, including physicians, nurses, and pharmacists, are more often addicted to drugs than are other people (that is, a higher percentage of health professionals has an addiction problem than does the general population).

If you or someone you work with becomes addicted to alcohol or other drugs, help is available. Most state pharmacy associations have some type of program for impaired pharmacists and technicians. While most people enter these programs after being caught stealing medications from the pharmacy workplace, some agree to enter treatment because their medication dependence is affecting their work performance. Additionally, if the state board of pharmacy becomes aware of the problem, the person's professional license may be revoked, and a condition of reinstatement may be successful completion of therapy in an impaired-health-professional program. Contact your state pharmacy association or the American Pharmacists Association at (800) 237-APHA or www.aphanet.org for more information.

If you or someone you work with becomes addicted to alcohol or other drugs, help is available. Most state pharmacy associations have some type of program for impaired pharmacists and technicians.

Conclusion

Formularies, storage, recalls, and diversion are concepts important to understanding contemporary pharmacy practice. Hopefully, this chapter has given you useful background information about each of these topics that you will find valuable in your job as a pharmacy technician. The next chapter presents another topic you will certainly hear about in the pharmacy—quality assurance.

For More Information

If you are preparing for the Pharmacy Technician Certification Examination and feel that you need more information about the topics discussed in this chapter, consider studying these sources of additional information:

- Desselle SP, Zgarrick DP. *Pharmacy Management: Essentials for All Practice Settings.* New York: McGraw-Hill; 2005:95–108.
- Peterson AM. *Managing Pharmacy Practice: Principles, Strategies, and Systems.* Boca Raton, Fla.: CRC Press; 2004.

References

American Society of Hospital Pharmacists. ASHP guidelines on formulary system management. *Am J Hosp Pharm.* 1992;49:648–52.

American Society of Hospital Pharmacists. ASHP technical assistance bulletin on drug formularies. *Am J Hosp Pharm.* 1991;48:791–3.

PART IV

Assisting with Pharmacy Administration and Management

CHAPTER FOURTEEN

Quality Assurance and Control

Pharmacy technicians play an important role in the overall operation and management of pharmacies. Chapter 14 will detail some of your roles and responsibilities in quality control and quality assurance.

Introduction

Quality, like beauty, is often in the eye of the beholder. What is considered high quality by one person might be completely unacceptable to the next person.

Within pharmacy and other parts of health care, customers—who, in a broad sense, might be physicians or nurses just as easily as patients—have a wide variety of expectations regarding the products involved and the services they expect. For pharmacy, products are usually medications and related devices. Services include the speed with which medications are provided and the information that is provided along with the product, as well as clinical services such as providing drug information to physicians and nurses, checking for drug interactions, monitoring for effectiveness and side effects, and referring patients to other providers when necessary.

Testing for variances in prescriptions and other work performed in the pharmacy falls under the broad framework known as quality assurance. Specific quality control tests are used to assess quality assurance. In this chapter, we focus on the quality assurance of pharmaceutical products because that is what you are most likely to be involved with in your role as a pharmacy technician. Be aware that when your pharmacy managers are attempting to measure service indicators—such as the time for prescriptions to be dispensed, contaminated intravenous solutions, prescription error rates, or out-of-stock frequencies—they are involved in the same process of quality assurance using quality control measures.

You will also hear people using the term quality improvement. This concept incorporates the philosophy that it is not enough to ensure quality; you should always seek to improve processes and systems so that quality continually improves. While not discussed specifically in this chapter, quality improvement is a desirable goal for both prescription processing and other more subjective measures of quality likely to be important to the "customers" of the pharmacy.

Principles of Quality Assurance and Control

Imagine that you own a factory that makes a toy ball. Inside each ball is a small doll, but the balls are sealed inside plastic wrapping when they come off the conveyor belt. Because children want to be able to pick out the ball with the correct doll inside, it is critically important that the package labeling match the contents of the ball. But, to check to see if the packaging has been matched correctly with the ball and its contents, you would have to open the package, thereby destroying the marketable product. How would you ensure the quality of the manufacturing process in this situation?

Well, you could take several approaches. Various checks could be put into the manufacturing process. Quality assurance of this process would start with only having the correct packaging and dolls present on the manufacturing line during production. Employees would double-check one another when the packaging, balls, and dolls are placed into the machine that combines them. Then, as a final check, a small percentage of the finished packages would be opened and checked to make sure they are correct. If any incorrect dolls or packages are found, then more packages would be opened to see if the problem is widespread. If more incorrect products are found, then the entire batch of products might be opened and repackaged correctly.

Those are the precise elements used in many pharmacies as means of quality assurance. If you review Chapter 5 and think about all the things that could go wrong at each step, you will have a good idea of the task confronting anyone seeking to ensure quality in the pharmacy. The major areas in which errors most often occur during prescription processing are discussed in Table 14-1.

TABLE 14-1

Errors in Prescription Processing

The major areas in which errors most often occur during prescription processing are:

- Incorrect interpretation of the prescription or medication order
- Incorrect entry of the order into the computer
- Incorrect medication, dosage form, or strength picked from storage shelves or bins
- Incorrect amount of medication placed in container
- Incorrect label attached to vial or product
- Incomplete or improper auxiliary labels attached to vial or product
- Prescription given to wrong patient

These errors occur in all pharmacy settings, with oral medications in the community, long-term care, and hospital pharmacy; with injectable medications in the hospital or home care pharmacy; and with compounded prescriptions in any pharmacy. However, there is an important difference between oral and injectable or compounded medications. With an oral medication in a prescription vial, you can check the color and markings on tablets and capsules to see if the correct drug was picked, and you can count the number of tablets. Thus, every prescription for oral medications you prepare can be checked by a pharmacist for accuracy. But with injectable or compounded products, visual inspection is usually impossible. Most injectable products are clear and colorless, regardless of how much drug was put in the solution. Compounded creams and ointments are usually the color and consistency of the base product, whether no drug or 10 times the proper amount was incorporated. To ensure quality for most injectable and compounded products, pharmacists must use techniques such as those described above for the toy factory.

The basis of any quality assurance system is proper training of personnel.

Importance of Training

The basis of any quality assurance system is proper training of personnel. For technicians who work in community pharmacies or unit-dose areas of hospitals and long-term care pharmacies, such training ensures that they are familiar with the drugs they prepare and that they understand pharmacy procedures. In the admixture room of the hospital, home care, or long-term care pharmacy, technicians must be familiar with the drugs as well as the principles of aseptic technique and sterile product preparation. For compounding, knowledge of the drug properties, available equipment, and correct techniques is required to obtain a high-quality product. All subsequent parts of the quality assurance process rest on a knowledgeable worker performing tasks in which he or she is competent.

Quality Control of Solid Oral Dosage Forms

For solid oral medications, the pharmacist will generally check every prescription or medication order processed by technicians. The pharmacist may ask you to keep out the container from which you obtained the medication to make sure it is the correct product.

FIGURE 14-1

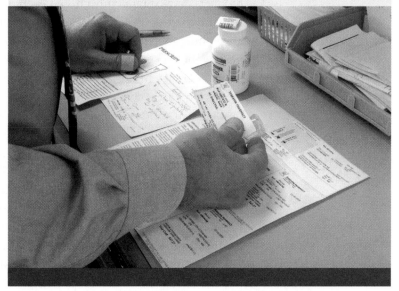

A pharmacist checks the work of a technician before dispensing a prescription.

As a pharmacy technician, especially in hospitals or other institutional pharmacies, you may be asked to help collect data for quality assurance programs.

The directions on the prescription label will be checked against the original physician's order (Figure 14-1). Many computer systems now have a scanned facsimile of the prescription that can be displayed on the screen. These systems also often have a picture of the correct tablet or capsule on the screen for the pharmacist to check against the product inside the vial (as seen in Figure 7-2). In some hi-tech pharmacies such as mail-service, very high-volume operations, computer systems use a small camera to electronically check the product inside the vial to make sure it matches the image stored in its files. The pharmacist will also look at the auxiliary labels you placed on the bottle. If everything is correct, the pharmacist dispenses (or authorizes to be dispensed) the prescription to the patient and provides any needed counseling about proper use of the medication.

In hospitals where solid oral dosage forms are placed into patient carts, a similar checking process is used. Because nurses check the medications again before giving them to patients, a few states allow technicians to check other technicians on cart fills, thereby freeing up the pharmacists' time for other activities. Most larger hospitals now have robotic devices that do most of the cart fills, and the bar-coding process used with robots ensures virtually 100% accuracy. No checks of the robot are generally done, but caution is required to be sure that the robot's bins were filled with the correct product.

Quality Control of Sterile and Nonsterile Compounded Products

In intravenous admixture and compounding areas, standard procedures will likely call for you to have nothing in the laminar-flow hood or preparation area except those items you are using to prepare the specific product. Pharmacists will check prescriptions individually, but the appearance of the product is not as helpful as with solid oral dosage forms. Rather, the pharmacist may ask you to keep all injectable product vials—empty or not—for inspection, generally with the syringe pulled back to the amount you put into the admixture. For certain types of admixtures, such as chemotherapy, total parenteral nutrition (TPN), and heparin, another technician or the pharmacist must check all calculations to be sure they are correct. Similar processes are used to check compounded prescriptions, including retaining all bulk containers and indicating how much of each ingredient you used.

Finally, the quality assurance system requires checking of a small percentage of admixtures and compounded products further, similar to opening the packages in the toy factory. For instance, to check for sterility of intravenous admixtures, a 2% sample of the outgoing products may be randomly chosen each day for testing of bacterial or fungal contamination. Because the tests often destroy the product, these units must sometimes be made again. If any contaminated samples are detected in this 2% sample, the percentage of sampled units may be increased temporarily to 5% or more. If further contaminated units are found, then the system may be declared "out of control," leading to a process of decontaminating the preparation area, checking the technique of personnel, and retraining employees when needed. This process and increased sampling would be continued until the system is back "in control," after which the 2% sampling would resume.

Similar chemical testing of TPN admixtures is also sometimes used. Samples of prepared units can be sent to the laboratory for analysis of pH (hydrogen ion concentration) and dextrose (sugar), amino acid, sodium, potassium, calcium, phosphate, and chloride content. In this case, the units are not destroyed, so higher percentages of units can be sampled (even up to 100% of units, if needed) at times when problems are occurring with product quality. If problems persist, pharmacy managers might correlate inaccurate units with certain personnel, products, or work shifts in an attempt to correct the system. However, they also need to check with laboratory managers, because errors can be made there as well.

Conclusion

As a pharmacy technician, especially in hospitals or other institutional pharmacies, you may be asked to help collect data for quality assurance programs. If so, the information in this chapter will help you understand how the data will be used in identifying and rectifying problems with quality in the pharmacy.

The final chapter is an overview of the pharmacy-specific policies and procedures that you need to review. Let's go to Chapter 15 to see what's involved.

For More Information

If you are preparing for the Pharmacy Technician Certification Examination and feel that you need more information about the topics discussed in this chapter, consider studying these sources of additional information:

- Peterson AM. Principles of inventory management. In: *Managing Pharmacy Practice: Principles, Strategies, and Systems.* Boca Raton, Fla.: CRC Press; 2004.
- Jackson TL. Ensuring quality in pharmacy operations. In: Desselle SP, Zgarrick DP. *Pharmacy Management: Essentials for All Practice Settings.* New York: McGraw-Hill; 2005:125–50.

References

American Society of Health-System Pharmacists. ASHP guidelines on the safe use of automated medication storage and distribution devices. *Am J Health Syst Pharm.* 1998;55:1403–7.

American Society of Hospital Pharmacists. ASHP technical assistance bulletin on quality assurance for pharmacy-prepared sterile products. *Am J Hosp Pharm.* 1993;50:2386–98.

American Society of Hospital Pharmacists. ASHP guidelines on preventing medication errors in hospitals. *Am J Hosp Pharm.* 1993;50:305–14.

CHAPTER FIFTEEN

Fitting into Your Workplace

Most of the third section of responsibilities outlined in the Pharmacy Technician Certification Examination Content Outline (see Appendix) are specific to your workplace and the policies and procedures that are used there. This final chapter wraps up the book by providing a summary of topics that technicians should discuss with their supervisors or employers.

Introduction

To succeed in your job as a pharmacy technician—and perhaps to turn it into your lifetime career—you must first be a successful employee and worker. To do this, you need to understand your role in the pharmacy, focus on accurately completing those tasks assigned to you, and contribute to the mission of the pharmacy and its professional and financial success.

In this chapter, we will look at how you can best contribute as a pharmacy technician. We will consider the topics that you need to learn about through your pharmacy's training sessions, policy and procedure manual, or managers.

Understanding Your Role as a Pharmacy Technician

A primary lesson to remember is that everyone must answer to someone else about his or her job. Even the president of the United States must account for his actions to the voters, to Congress, to the courts, and to other leaders around the world. Likewise, everyone in a company or business reports to someone with respect to his or her actions. Even the owner must account to the customers or governmental authorities in certain situations.

As a pharmacy technician, you should keep in mind the role you play. While you may be responsible for preparing prescription medications for patients, the pharmacist must ultimately bear responsibility for the accuracy of your work. From a management perspective, managers and pharmacists attempt to ensure the accuracy of prescriptions and the overall success of the pharmacy through five functions, as discussed in Table 15-1.

Keep in mind that the managers, supervisors, and pharmacists with whom you work have expected duties they must perform in these five areas. To be a successful employee, you need to understand what you are expected to do (job description), when and how tasks are to be completed (either through verbal instructions from supervisors or policy and procedure manuals), and how you can help gather data to show that the desired quality and outcomes are being attained. In addition, if a manager or supervisor is "checking up on you," remember that it is his or her job to do so. Further, if the pharmacist is "looking over your shoulder," remember that he or she bears both legal and ethical responsibility for your actions—and that the two of you will either succeed or fail together. The two of you are in the same boat, and it is in both your and the pharmacist's best interest to work together (Figure 15-1).

Pharmacy interns may be employed in your pharmacy on occasion, or you may encounter student pharmacists who are on rotations. These pharmacists-in-training may be performing duties similar to yours, or they may be used in specific ways that relate to the areas of study they are emphasizing in this particular pharmacy. When they are in your area, talk with them about what they expect to learn and help them to achieve their educational goals. Interns and student pharmacists are generally not licensed as pharmacists, and prescriptions they have prepared must be checked by the pharmacist before dispensing.

TABLE 15-1

Five Functions for Pharmacy Success

Managers and pharmacists attempt to ensure the accuracy of prescriptions and the overall success of the pharmacy by using these functions:

- **Planning** — Setting the mission, short- and long-term goals, processes, and procedures that guide workers in the pharmacy
- **Organizing** — Establishing job descriptions and defining the relationships among various workers
- **Staffing** — Hiring people into positions who have the necessary qualifications for the expected duties
- **Directing** — Communicating with staff about when and how tasks are to be completed and providing the needed motivation and leadership
- **Controlling** — Checking on quality and outcomes to make sure that staff actions and pharmacy processes are resulting in the desired products and services

Following Policies and Procedures

Like most small businesses, independent community pharmacies rarely have extensive orientation sessions for new employees, policy and procedure manuals, or employee handbooks. But it is just as important for you to obtain this information as it is in hospitals, health systems, and national chain or long-term care pharmacies.

During orientation sessions, basic employment information (especially benefits and company policies about sickness, vacation, and insurance) is usually presented. Ideally, this information will be contained in an employee handbook, as much of it may not be relevant to you at this point in your employment. An employee handbook typically contains sections on the subjects listed in Table 15-2.

In larger pharmacies and organizations, formal training sessions may be provided as well. These may last several weeks or months and are often combined with on-the-job training. Many pharmacy technicians gain their knowledge about pharmacy through these sessions.

The policy and procedure manual guides much activity in the pharmacy, and this information may be presented at orientation or training sessions. If your pharmacy does not have a manual, you will still need to make sure that you understand what to do in many situations. Make sure that you have the information you need about each. If not, consult the manual or talk with your supervisor.

An important subject to check into early in your employment is company policy about performance reviews and salary and promotion reviews. You may be on "probation" for a few months at the beginning of your employment, with monthly reviews of your progress. Be sure to take advantage of these opportunities to talk with your supervisor about how you are doing and about any problems you have encountered in your job. After the probation period, you will likely have only one scheduled chance each year to get formal feedback and to talk privately with your supervisor.

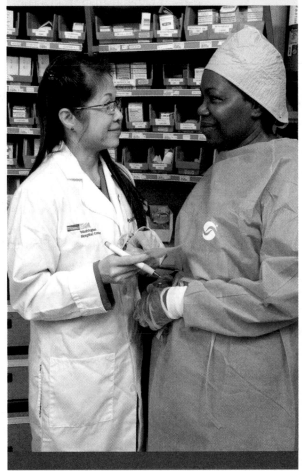

FIGURE 15-1

A hospital pharmacist and technician discussing their work.

TABLE 15-2

The Employee Handbook

An employee handbook typically contains sections on these subjects:

- History, mission, goals, and objectives of the pharmacy or organization
- Operating hours, rest and lunch periods, absences, pay periods, shift premiums, safety and accident prevention, use of computers (including the Internet and e-mail) and telephones for personal communication

- Benefits, including vacation, sick leave, life and medical insurance, parking, savings plans, payment of employee expenses (association dues, continuing education sessions), jury duty and military leave, and unemployment compensation
- Other information, including discounts on purchases, education benefits, and company activities (holiday parties, sports leagues, picnics)

Conclusion

Most people spend more waking hours at work than they do with their families. Employment establishes a special relationship between the company and the employees, and special friendships often develop among employees. By understanding the information usually found in the employee handbook and policy and procedure manual, you can give yourself the best chances of success in your job as a pharmacy technician.

For More Information

If you are preparing for the Pharmacy Technician Certification Examination and feel that you need more information about the topics discussed in this chapter, consider studying these sources of additional information:

- Review the PTCB responsibility and knowledge items listed under Section 3, Participating in the Administration and Management of Pharmacy Practice, in Appendix A, and look for the related information in your employer's policy and procedure manual or talk with your supervisor about these items.
- Snipe K. Pharmacy technician job description and duties. In: *The Pharmacy Technician Skills-Building Manual*. Washington, D.C.: American Pharmacists Association; 2007:1-8.

Appendices

This section lists the responsibilities and knowledge students must master as they prepare for the Pharmacy Technician Certification Examination, and notes where the subject matter is covered in this text.

Percentage Distribution of the Pharmacy Technician Certification Examination

FUNCTION		PERCENTAGE OF EXAMINATION ITEMS
01	**Assisting the Pharmacist in Serving Patients** Activities related to prescription/medication order preparation and dispensing; medication provision and administration; the collection, organization, and dissemination of information related to individual patients; and communication with third-party payers. Includes regulatory and quality assurance mechanisms associated with these activities.	66
02	**Maintaining Medication and Inventory Control Systems** Activities related to the purchasing, inventory control, storage and handling, and preparation and distribution of medications, durable and non-durable medical equipment, and supplies. Includes regulatory and quality assurance mechanisms associated with these activities.	22
03	**Participating in the Administration and Management of Pharmacy Practice** Activities related to the administration, operations, and management processes for the pharmacy practice site including quality assurance, accounting, human resources, facilities, equipment, and information systems.	12
TOTAL		100

Responsibilities Tested in the PTCB Examination

I   Assisting the Pharmacist in Serving Patients (66% of examination items)

RESPONSIBILITY		CHAPTER(S) IN THIS BOOK COVERING RESPONSIBILITY
A	Receive prescription/medication order(s) from patient/patient's representative, prescriber, or other healthcare professional	
	1 Accept new prescription/medication order from patient/patient's representative, prescriber, or other healthcare professional	5
	2 Accept new prescription/medication order electronically (for example, by telephone, fax, or electronic transmission)	5
	3 Accept refill request from patient/patient's representative	5
	4 Accept refill authorization from prescriber or other healthcare professional electronically (for example, by telephone, fax, or electronic transmission)	5
	5 Contact prescriber/originator for clarification of prescription/medication order refill	5
	6 Perform/accept transfer of prescription/medication order(s)	5
B	Assist the pharmacist in accordance with federal rules and regulations in obtaining from the patient/patient's representative such information as diagnosis or desired therapeutic outcome, disease state, medication history (including over-the-counter [OTC] medications and dietary supplements), allergies, adverse reactions, medical history and other relevant patient information, physical disability, and payer information (including both self-pay and third-party reimbursement)	4, 5, 8, 11
C	Assist the pharmacist in accordance with federal rules and regulations in obtaining from prescriber, other healthcare professionals, and/or the medical record such information as diagnosis or desired therapeutic outcome, disease state, medication history (including over-the-counter [OTC] medications and dietary supplements), allergies, adverse reactions, medical history and other relevant patient information, physical disability, and payer information (including both self-pay and third-party reimbursement)	4, 5, 11
D	Collect and communicate patient-specific data (for example, blood pressure, glucose, cholesterol levels, therapeutic drug levels, immunizations) to assist the pharmacist in monitoring patient outcomes	6
E	Collect and communicate data related to restricted drug distribution programs (for example, thalidomide, isotretinoin, clozapine)	3, 4
F	Collect and communicate data related to investigational drugs	3
G	Assess prescription or medication order for completeness (for example, patient's name and address), accuracy, authenticity, legality, and reimbursement eligibility	4, 5, 11
H	Update the medical record/patient profile with such information as medication history (including [OTC] medications and dietary supplements), disease states, compliance/adherence patterns, allergies, medication duplication, and/or drug–disease, drug–drug, drug–laboratory, drug–dietary supplement and/or OTC, and drug–food interactions	4, 6, 7
I	Assist the patient/patient's representative in choosing the best payment assistance plan if multiple plans are available to patient	11

Responsibilities Tested in the PTCB Examination

RESPONSIBILITY		CHAPTER(S) IN THIS BOOK COVERING RESPONSIBILITY
J	Process a prescription/medication order	
1	Enter prescription/medication order information into patient profile	4, 5
2	Select the appropriate product(s) for dispensing (for example, brand names, generic substitutes, therapeutic substitutes, formulary restrictions)	4, 5
3	Obtain pharmaceuticals, durable and non-durable medical equipment, devices, and supplies (including hazardous substances, controlled substances, and investigational products) from inventory	4, 5
4	Calculate quantity and days supply of finished dosage forms for dispensing	2
5	Measure or count quantity of finished dosage forms for dispensing	3
6	Process and handle radiopharmaceuticals	10
7	Perform calculations for radiopharmaceuticals	2
8	Process and handle chemotherapeutic medications commercially available in finished dosage forms (for example, Efudex, mercaptopurine)	10
9	Perform calculations for oral chemotherapeutic medications	2
10	Process and handle investigational products	3
11	Package finished dosage forms (for example, blister pack, robotic/automated dispensing, vial)	5
12	Affix label(s) and auxiliary label(s) to container(s)	5
13	Assemble patient information materials (for example, drug information sheets, patient package inserts, Health Insurance Portability and Accountability Act [HIPAA] literature)	5
14	Check for accuracy during processing of the prescription/medication order (for example, National Drug Code [NDC] number, bar code, and data entry)	5
15	Verify the data entry, measurements, preparation, and/or packaging of medications produced by other technicians as allowed by law (for example, tech check tech)	5
16	Prepare prescription or medication order for final check by pharmacist	5
17	Prepare prescription or medication order for final check by pharmacy technician as allowed by law (for example, tech check tech)	5
18	Perform Nuclear Regulatory Commission (NRC) required checks for radiopharmaceuticals	10

Responsibilities Tested in the PTCB Examination

RESPONSIBILITY			CHAPTER(S) IN THIS BOOK COVERING RESPONSIBILITY
K		Compound a prescription/medication order	
	1	Assemble equipment and/or supplies necessary for compounding the prescription/medication order	9, 10
	2	Calibrate equipment (for example, scale or balance, total parenteral nutrition [TPN] compounder) needed to compound the prescription/medication order	9, 10
	3	Perform calculations required for preparation of compounded IV admixtures	2, 10
	4	Perform calculations for extemporaneous compounds	2, 9, 10
	5	Compound medications (for example, topical preparations, reconstituted antibiotic suspensions) for dispensing according to prescription and/or compounding guidelines	9, 10
	6	Compound medications in anticipation of prescriptions/medication orders (for example, compounding for a specific patient)	9, 10
	7	Prepare sterile products (for example, TPNs, piggybacks, IV solutions, ophthalmic products)	10
	8	Prepare radiopharmaceuticals	10
	9	Prepare chemotherapy	10
	10	Record preparation and/or ingredients of medications (for example, lot number, control number, expiration date, chemotherapy calculations, type of IV solution)	9, 10
L		Provide prescription/medication to patient/patient's representative	
	1	Store medication prior to distribution	8
	2	Provide medication and supplemental information (for example, patient package inserts) to patient/patient's representative	5, 8
	3	Package and ship pharmaceuticals, durable and non-durable medical equipment, devices, and supplies (including hazardous substances and investigational products) to patient/patient's representative	8
	4	Place medication in dispensing system (for example, unit-dose cart, automated systems)	8
	5	Deliver medication to patient-care unit	8
	6	Record distribution of prescription medication	8
	7	Record distribution of controlled substances	8
	8	Record distribution of investigational drugs	8
	9	Record distribution of restricted drugs (for example, isotretinoin, clozapine, thalidomide)	8
	10	Record distribution of prescription/medication to patient's home	8
M		Determine charges and obtain reimbursement for products and services	11

Responsibilities Tested in the PTCB Examination

RESPONSIBILITY			CHAPTER(S) IN THIS BOOK COVERING RESPONSIBILITY
	N	Communicate with third-party payers to determine or verify coverage	11
	O	Communicate with third-party payers to obtain prior authorizations	11
	P	Communicate with third-party payers and patients/patient's representatives to rectify rejected third-party claims	11
	Q	Identify and resolve problems with rejected claims (for example, incorrect days supply, incorrect ID number)	2
	R	Provide supplemental information (for example, disease-state information, CDs) as requested/required	11
	S	Direct patient/patient's representative to pharmacist for counseling	8
	T	Perform drug administration functions under appropriate supervision (for example, perform drug/IV rounds, check pumps, anticipate refill of drugs/IVs)	10
	U	Process and dispense enteral products	9, 10

II Maintaining Medication and Inventory Control Systems (22% of examination items)

	A	Identify pharmaceuticals, durable and non-durable medical equipment, devices, and supplies (including hazardous substances and investigational products) to be ordered	12
	B	Place routine orders for pharmaceuticals, durable and non-durable medical equipment, devices, and supplies (including hazardous substances and investigational products) in compliance with legal, regulatory, formulary, budgetary, and contractual requirements	12 / 12
	C	Place emergency orders for pharmaceuticals, durable and non-durable medical equipment, devices, and supplies (including hazardous substances and investigational products) in compliance with legal, regulatory, formulary, budgetary, and contractual requirements	12
	D	Receive pharmaceuticals, durable and non-durable medical equipment, devices, and supplies (including hazardous substances and investigational products) and verify against specifications on original purchase orders	12
	E	Place pharmaceuticals, durable and non-durable medical equipment, devices, and supplies (including hazardous substances and investigational products) in inventory under proper storage conditions while incorporating error prevention strategies	12
	F	Perform non–patient-specific preparation, distribution, and maintenance of pharmaceuticals, durable and non-durable medical equipment, devices, and supplies (including hazardous substances and investigational products) while incorporating error prevention strategies (for example, crash carts, clinic and nursing floor stock, automated dispensing systems)	14
	G	Remove from inventory expired/discontinued/slow-moving/overstocked pharmaceuticals, durable and non-durable medical equipment, devices, and supplies (including hazardous substances and investigational products)	13
	H	Remove from inventory recalled pharmaceuticals, durable and non-durable medical equipment, devices, and supplies (including hazardous substances and investigational products)	13
	I	Dispose of or destroy pharmaceuticals or supplies (for example, hazardous substances, investigational products, controlled substances, non-dispensable products)	13
	J	Communicate changes in product availability (for example, formulary changes, recalls, shortages) to pharmacy staff, patient/patient's representative, physicians, and other healthcare professionals	15

Responsibilities Tested in the PTCB Examination

RESPONSIBILITY		CHAPTER(S) IN THIS BOOK COVERING RESPONSIBILITY
K	Implement and monitor policies and procedures to deter theft and/or drug diversion	13
L	Maintain a record of controlled substances ordered, received, and removed from inventory	13
M	Maintain a record of investigational products ordered, received, and removed from inventory	13
N	Perform required inventories and maintain associated records	13
O	Maintain record-keeping systems for repackaging, non-patient specific compounding, recalls, and returns of pharmaceuticals, durable and non-durable medical equipment, devices, and supplies (including hazardous substances and investigational products)	12
P	Compound non–patient-specific medications in anticipation of prescription/medication orders	9
Q	Perform quality assurance tests on compounded medications (for example, end product testing and validation)	9, 10, 14
R	Repackage finished dosage forms for dispensing (for example, unit dose, blister pack, oral syringes)	9

III Participating in the Administration and Management of Pharmacy Practice (12% of examination items)

A	Coordinate written, electronic, and oral communications throughout the practice setting (for example, route phone calls, faxes, verbal and written refill authorizations; disseminate policy and procedure changes)	15
B	Update and maintain patient information (for example, insurance information, demographics, provider information) in accordance with federal regulations and professional standards (for example, Health Insurance Portability and Accountability Act [HIPAA])	8
C	Collect productivity information (for example, the number of prescriptions filled, fill times, payments collected, rejected claim status)	15
D	Participate in quality assurance activities (for example, medication error prevention, customer satisfaction surveys, internal audits of processes)	14
E	Generate quality assurance reports (for example, compile or summarize data collected for evaluation or action plan development, root cause analysis)	14
F	Implement and monitor the practice setting for compliance with federal regulations and professional standards (for example, Material Safety Data Sheet [MSDS], Occupational Safety and Health Administration [OSHA], Joint Commission on Accreditation of Healthcare Organizations [JCAHO], United States Pharmacopeia [USP])	3
G	Implement and monitor policies and procedures for infection control	10
H	Implement and monitor policies and procedures for the handling, disposal, and destruction of pharmaceuticals and supplies (for example, hazardous substances, investigational products, controlled substances, non-dispensable products, radiopharmaceuticals)	13
I	Perform and record routine sanitation, maintenance, and calibration of equipment (for example, automated dispensing equipment, balances, TPN compounders, refrigerator/freezer temperatures)	9, 10, 14
J	Update, maintain, and use manual or electronic information systems (for example, patient profiles, prescription records, inventory logs, reference materials) in order to perform job-related activities	7
K	Use and maintain automated and point-of-care dispensing technology	7

Responsibilities Tested in the PTCB Examination

RESPONSIBILITY			CHAPTER(S) IN THIS BOOK COVERING RESPONSIBILITY
	L	Perform billing and accounting functions for products and services (for example, self-pay, third-party adjudication, pharmaceutical discount cards, medication reimbursement)	11
	M	Communicate with third-party payers to determine or verify coverage for products and services	11
	N	Coordinate and/or participate in staff training and continuing education	15
	O	Perform and/or contribute to employee evaluations and competency assessments	15
	P	Participate in the establishment, implementation, and monitoring of the practice setting's policies and procedures	15

Knowledge Base Required to Perform Responsibilities Associated with Each Function of Pharmacy Technicians

FUNCTION I   ASSISTING THE PHARMACIST IN SERVING PATIENTS

KNOWLEDGE OF:		CHAPTER(S) IN THIS BOOK COVERING RESPONSIBILITY
1	Federal, state, and/or practice site regulations, codes of ethics, and standards pertaining to the practice of pharmacy	3
2	Pharmaceutical, medical, and legal developments which impact the practice of pharmacy	3
3	State-specific prescription transfer regulations	3
4	Pharmaceutical and medical abbreviations and terminology	2, 5
5	Generic and brand names of pharmaceuticals	4, 5
6	Therapeutic equivalence	3
7	Epidemiology	4
8	Risk factors for disease	4
9	Anatomy and physiology	4
10	Signs and symptoms of disease states	4
11	Standard and abnormal laboratory values	4
12	Drug interactions (such as drug–disease, drug–drug, drug–dietary supplement, drug–OTC, drug–laboratory, drug–nutrient)	4
13	Strengths/dose, dosage forms, physical appearance, routes of administration, and duration of drug therapy	4
14	Effects of patient's age (for example, neonates, geriatrics) on drug and non-drug therapy	4
15	Drug information sources including printed and electronic reference materials	4, 8
16	Pharmacology (for example, mechanism of action)	4
17	Common and severe side or adverse effects, allergies, and therapeutic contraindications associated with medications	4
18	Drug indications	4
19	Relative role of drug and non-drug therapy (for example, dietary supplementation, lifestyle modification, smoking cessation)	4
20	Practice site policies and procedures regarding prescriptions or medication orders	15
21	Information to be obtained from patient/patient's representative (for example, demographic information, allergy, third-party information)	5
22	Required prescription order refill information	5
23	Formula to verify the validity of a prescriber's DEA number	3
24	Techniques for detecting forged or altered prescriptions	3
25	Techniques for detecting prescription errors (for example, abnormal doses, early refill, incorrect quantity, incorrect patient ID #, incorrect drug)	3, 5
26	Effects of patient disabilities (for example, visual, physical) on drug and non-drug therapy	5
27	Techniques, equipment, and supplies for drug administration (for example, insulin syringes and IV tubing)	10
28	Non-prescription (over-the-counter [OTC]) formulations	4

Knowledge Base Required to Perform Responsibilities Associated with Each Function of Pharmacy Technicians

FUNCTION I   ASSISTING THE PHARMACIST IN SERVING PATIENTS

KNOWLEDGE OF:		CHAPTER(S) IN THIS BOOK COVERING RESPONSIBILITY
29	Monitoring and screening equipment (for example, blood pressure cuffs, glucose monitors)	6
30	Medical and surgical appliances and devices (for example, ostomies, orthopedic devices, pumps)	6
31	Proper storage conditions	13
32	Automated dispensing technology	7
33	Packaging requirements	9
34	NDC number components	3
35	Purpose for lot numbers and expiration dates	3, 13
36	Information for prescription or medication order label(s)	5
37	Requirements regarding auxiliary labels	5
38	Requirements regarding patient package inserts	5
39	Special directions and precautions for patient/patient's representative regarding preparation and use of medications	8
40	Techniques for assessing patient's compliance with prescription or medication order	8
41	Action to be taken in the event of a missed dose	8
42	Requirements for mailing medications	3
43	Delivery systems for distributing medications (for example, pneumatic tube, robotics)	7
44	Requirements for dispensing controlled substances	3
45	Requirements for dispensing investigational drugs	3
46	Record-keeping requirements for medication dispensing	3
47	Automatic stop orders	13
48	Restricted drug programs	13
49	Quality improvement methods (for example, matching NDC number, double-counting narcotics)	14
50	Calculations (for example, algebra, ratio and proportions, metric conversions, IV drip rates, IV admixture calculations)	2
51	Measurement systems (for example, metric and avoirdupois)	2
52	Drug stability	10
53	Physical and chemical incompatibilities	10
54	Equipment calibration techniques	10
55	Procedures to prepare IV admixtures	10
56	Procedures to prepare chemotherapy	10
57	Procedures to prepare total parenteral nutrition (TPN) solutions	10
58	Procedures to prepare reconstituted injectable and non-injectable medications	9, 10

Knowledge Base Required to Perform Responsibilities Associated with Each Function of Pharmacy Technicians

FUNCTION I   ASSISTING THE PHARMACIST IN SERVING PATIENTS

KNOWLEDGE OF:		CHAPTER(S) IN THIS BOOK COVERING RESPONSIBILITY
59	Specialized procedures to prepare injectable medications (for example, epidurals and patient controlled analgesic [PCA] cassettes)	10
60	Procedures to prepare radiopharmaceuticals	10
61	Procedures to prepare oral dosage forms (for example, tablets, capsules, liquids) in unit-dose or non–unit-dose packaging	9
62	Procedures to compound sterile non-injectable products (for example, eye drops)	10
63	Procedures to compound non-sterile products (for example, ointments, mixtures, liquids, emulsions)	9
64	Procedures to prepare ready-to-dispense multidose packages (for example, ophthalmics, otics, inhalers, topicals, transdermals)	9
65	Aseptic techniques (for example, laminar flow hood, filters)	10
66	Infection control procedures	10
67	Requirements for handling hazardous products and disposing of hazardous waste	10
68	Documentation requirements for controlled substances, investigational drugs, and hazardous wastes	3
69	Pharmacy-related computer software for documenting the dispensing of prescriptions or medication orders	5, 7
70	Manual systems for documenting the dispensing of prescriptions or medication orders	5
71	Customer service principles	8
72	Communication techniques	8
73	Confidentiality requirements	8
74	Cash handling procedures	8
75	Reimbursement policies and plans	11
76	Legal requirements for pharmacist counseling of patient/patient's representative	3, 8

FUNCTION II   MAINTAINING MEDICATION AND INVENTORY CONTROL SYSTEMS

KNOWLEDGE OF:		CHAPTER(S) IN THIS BOOK COVERING RESPONSIBILITY
1	Drug product laws and regulations and professional standards related to obtaining medication supplies, durable medical equipment, and products (for example, Food, Drug and Cosmetic Act; Controlled Substances Act; Prescription Drug Marketing Act; USP-NF; NRC standards)	3, 12
2	Pharmaceutical industry procedures for obtaining pharmaceuticals	12
3	Purchasing policies, procedures, and practices	12
4	Dosage forms	4

Knowledge Base Required to Perform Responsibilities
Associated with Each Function of Pharmacy Technicians

FUNCTION II MAINTAINING MEDICATION AND INVENTORY CONTROL SYSTEMS

KNOWLEDGE OF:		CHAPTER(S) IN THIS BOOK COVERING RESPONSIBILITY
5	Formulary or approved stock list	12, 13
6	Par and reorder levels and drug usage	12
7	Inventory receiving process	12
8	Bioavailability standards (for example, generic substitutes)	3
9	The use of DEA controlled substance ordering forms	3
10	Regulatory requirements regarding record-keeping for repackaged products, recalled products, and refunded products	3
11	Policies, procedures, and practices for inventory systems	12
12	Products used in packaging and repackaging (for example, child-resistant caps and light-protective unit-dose packaging)	5, 9
13	Risk management opportunities (for example, dress code, personal protective equipment [PPE], needle recapping)	10
14	The FDA's recall classifications	3, 13
15	Systems to identify and return expired and unsalable products	3, 13
16	Rules and regulations for the removal and disposal of products	3, 13
17	Legal and regulatory requirements and professional standards governing operations of pharmacies (for example, prepackaging, difference between compounding and manufacturing)	3, 9
18	Legal and regulatory requirements and professional standards (for example, FDA, DEA, state board of pharmacy, JCAHO) for preparing, labeling, dispensing, distributing, and administering medications	3, 5
19	Medication distribution and control systems requirements for the use of medications in various practice settings (for example, automated dispensing systems, bar coding, nursing stations, crash carts)	3, 12
20	Preparation, storage requirements, and documentation for medications compounded in anticipation of prescriptions or medication orders	9
21	Repackaging, storage requirements, and documentation for finished dosage forms prepared in anticipation of prescriptions or medication orders	9
22	Policies, procedures, and practices regarding storage and handling of hazardous substances and wastes (for example, Material Safety Data Sheet [MSDS])	3
23	Medication distribution and control systems requirements for controlled substances, investigational drugs, and hazardous substances and wastes	3
24	The written, oral, and electronic communication channels necessary to ensure appropriate follow-up and problem resolution (for example, product recalls, supplier shorts)	13
25	Quality assurance policies, procedures, and practices for medication and inventory control systems	14

Knowledge Base Required to Perform Responsibilities Associated with Each Function of Pharmacy Technicians

FUNCTION III PARTICIPATING IN THE ADMINISTRATION AND MANAGEMENT OF PHARMACY PRACTICE

KNOWLEDGE OF:		CHAPTER(S) IN THIS BOOK COVERING RESPONSIBILITY
1	The practice setting's mission, goals and objectives, organizational structure, and policies and procedures	15
2	Lines of communication throughout the organization	15
3	Principles of resource allocation (for example, budgeting, scheduling, cross training, work flow)	15
4	Productivity, efficiency, and customer satisfaction measures	15
5	Written, oral, and electronic communication systems	15
6	Required operational licenses and certificates	3
7	Roles and responsibilities of pharmacists, pharmacy technicians, and other pharmacy employees	1, 15
8	Legal and regulatory requirements for personnel, facilities, equipment, and supplies (for example, space requirements, prescription file storage, cleanliness, reference materials, storage of radiopharmaceuticals)	3, 15
9	Professional standards (for example, JCAHO) for personnel, facilities, equipment, and supplies	3, 15
10	Quality assurance standards and guidelines	15
11	State board of pharmacy regulations	3, 15
12	Storage requirements and expiration dates for equipment and supplies (for example, first-aid items, fire extinguishers)	15
13	Storage and handling requirements for hazardous substances (for example, chemotherapeutics, radiopharmaceuticals)	15
14	Hazardous waste disposal requirements	15
15	Procedures for the treatment of exposure to hazardous substances (for example, eyewash)	15
16	Security systems for the protection of employees, customers, and property	15
17	Laminar flow hood maintenance requirements	15
18	Infection control policies and procedures	15
19	Sanitation requirements (for example, handwashing, cleaning counting trays, countertop, and equipment)	15
20	Equipment maintenance and calibration	15
21	Supply procurement procedures	15
22	Technology used in the preparation, delivery, and administration of medications (for example, robotics, Baker cells, automated TPN equipment, Pyxis, infusion pumps)	7, 15
23	Purpose and function of pharmacy equipment	15
24	Documentation requirements for routine sanitation, maintenance, and equipment calibration	15
25	The Americans with Disabilities Act requirements (for example, physical limitations)	3
26	Manual and computer-based systems for storing, retrieving, and using pharmacy-related information (for example, drug interactions, patient profiles, generating labels)	7, 15
27	Security procedures related to data integrity, security, and confidentiality	15

Knowledge Base Required to Perform Responsibilities
Associated with Each Function of Pharmacy Technicians

FUNCTION III PARTICIPATING IN THE ADMINISTRATION AND MANAGEMENT OF PHARMACY PRACTICE

KNOWLEDGE OF:

		CHAPTER(S) IN THIS BOOK COVERING RESPONSIBILITY
28	Downtime emergency policies and procedures	15
29	Backup and archiving procedures for stored data and documentation	15
30	Legal requirements regarding archiving	15
31	Third-party reimbursement systems	11
32	Healthcare reimbursement systems (for example, home health, respiratory medications, eligibility and reimbursement)	11
33	Billing and accounting policies and procedures	15
34	Information sources used to obtain data in a quality improvement system (for example, the patient's chart, patient profile, computerized information systems, medication administration record)	15
35	Procedures to document occurrences such as medication errors, adverse events, and product integrity (for example, FDA MedWatch Program)	3, 15
36	Staff training techniques	15
37	Employee performance evaluation techniques	15
38	Employee performance feedback techniques	15

Index

A

Abbreviations
  adverse effects, 101t
  commonly used medications, 101t
  pharmaceutical, 21, 22t
Absorption of medication, 69–70, 69f
Abuse of Medicare and Medicaid, 174
Academy of Managed Care Pharmacy, 41
Accreditation, voluntary. *See also* Certification
  certification of individuals, 42, 42t
  reimbursement plans, 41
  training programs, 41–42
ACE (angiotensin-converting enzyme) inhibitors, 83t
Addiction, 196–197
Adulterated products, 30
Adverse effects
  abbreviations for, 101t
  described, 73t
Alkylating agents, 95t
Allergies, 73t
Alpha particles, 167
Alzheimer's disease, medications for, 77t
American Council on Pharmaceutical Education, 5
American Medical Association, 73t
American Pharmaceutical (Pharmacists) Association (APhA)
  addiction, 197
  code of ethics, 44f
  generic names, 73t
  pharmacy specialties, 120
  Pharmacy Technician Certification Board, 6
  state boards of pharmacy, 40, 41
American Pharmaceutical (Pharmacists) Association (APhA) Foundation, 122
American Society of Health-System Pharmacists
  Pharmacy Technician Certification Board, 6
  residency accreditation, 41, 42
Americans with Disabilities Act, 39–40, 40t
Analgesics
  centrally acting, 77t
  migraine, for, 78t
  musculoskeletal system, for, 88t
Anatomy, 51–65
  cardiovascular system, 60f, 62
  digestive system, 63–64, 63f, 64f
  endocrine system, 59, 59f, 62
  integumentary system, 53, 53f
  lymphatic system, 61f, 62–63
  muscular system, 55–56f, 58
  nervous system, 57f, 58–59, 58f
  organ systems, 51, 52t, 53
  reproductive system, 65, 66f
  respiratory system, 62f, 63
  skeletal system, 53, 54f
  urinary system, 64–65, 65f

Angiotensin-converting enzyme (ACE) inhibitors, 83t
Angiotensin receptor blockers (ARBs), 83t
Angry patients, 144t
Anterooms, 163, 164
Anti-infective agents, 90–94t, 99t. *See also* Antibiotics
Antiadrenergic agents, 84–85t
Antianxiety agents, 74t
Antibiotics
  chemotherapy, 97t
  commonly used, 90–92t
  stop orders, 193
  suspensions, preparing, 112f, 113–114
Anticoagulant agents, 86t
Antidepressants, 75t
Antiemetics, 78–79t
Antiepileptic medications, 78t
Antifungal agents, 92t
Antihistamines, 79t
Antihyperlipidemic agents, 85–86t
Antimetabolites, 96t
Antimitotic agents, 96t
Antiparkinsonian agents, 76–77t
Antiplatelet agents, 86t
Antipsychotic agents, 76t
Antiviral agents, 93–94t
Anxiolytics, 74t
Apothecary system, 11, 12t, 13t
ARBs (angiotensin receptor blockers), 83t
Aseptic technique
  procedures for, 161–165, 162t, 163f, 164f, 164t
  sterile compounding, 158, 159f, 164–165
Asheville Project, 122
Atoms
  chemical physiology, 48t, 49, 49f
  radiopharmaceuticals, 166
Attention-deficit/hyperactivity disorder, medications for, 78t
Automated cart-fill machines, 135
Automated point-of-care dispensing machines, 135–136
Automated prescription-dispensing systems, 135, 135f
Avoirdupois system, 11, 11t, 13t

B

Bachelor of Science (B.S.) in pharmacy, 5
Bacteria, 158, 159f
Bar-coding of inventory, 187, 187f, 188, 189
Benzodiazepines, 74t
Beta-agonists, 80t
Beta-blockers, 84t
Beta particles, 167
Beyond-use dates. *See* Expiration dates (beyond-use dates)

Computer systems
   confidentiality, 137
   inventory management, 187, 188, 188f, 189
   medication therapy management, 136, 137t
   pharmacy dispensing, 134–136, 134f, 135f, 135t
"Conditions of participation" in Medicare and
   Medicaid, 35
Confidentiality/privacy
   computerized systems, 137
   interactions with patients, 146–147
   obtaining information from patients, 109
Consumer Healthcare Products Association, 34
Containers
   nonsterile compounding, 152t, 153
   prescriptions, processing, 114–116, 114f, 115f
Contamination, 113. *See also* Aseptic technique
Contraindications to medication, 73t
Controlled clinical trials, 30, 31
Controlled substances
   categories of, 36, 36t
   DEA regulations, 35, 36–38, 36t, 37f
   inventory management, 189
   medication orders for, 108
   medication refills, 109t
   ordering, 36, 37f
   prescriptions for, 36–38
   storage of medications, 193
   theft, 195, 195f, 196–197
Controlled Substances Act of 1970, 35
Corticosteroids
   dermatologic, 100t
   endocrinologic uses, 82t
   inhaled, 80t
   nasal, 79t
Costs of inventory, 186, 186t
Costs of medical care, 122
Counting trays/devices, 112–113, 113f
COX-2 inhibitors, 88t
CPT (Common Procedural Terminology) codes,
   177t, 180, 180t, 181t
Creams, 52t
Credit for expired drug products, 193–194
Cytochrome P450 enzymes, 70, 102

D

DEA. *See* Drug Enforcement Administration
   (DEA)
Decoding messages, 140–141
Demographic information, 7, 7f
Depressed patients, 144t
Dermatologic agents, 99–100t
Diabetes, medications for, 81t
Diagnosis-related groups (DRGs), 174
Dialysis, peritoneal, 130
Dietary Supplement Health Education Act of
   1994, 32–33, 33t, 144

Dietary supplements, 143f, 144
Digestive system. *See* Gastroenterologic system
Direct payment for prescriptions, 172
Direct questions, 141t
Directions for Clinical Practice in Pharmacy con-
   ference, 120
Disabled persons, 39–40, 40t
Disease
   process of, 67
   risk factors for, 67–68, 69
   signs and symptoms, 68
"Dispense As Written," 110
Dissolution, 152
Distribution of medication, 70
Diversion of medications, 196–197
Doctor of pharmacy degree, 5
Dosage forms of medications, 51–52t, 72, 73t
Double blinded studies, 32
DRGs (diagnosis-related groups), 174
Drug-approval process, FDA, 30–32, 31f
Drug classifications and formulations. *See also*
   Anatomy; Medications
   anti-infective agents, 90–94t
   bone and joint agents, 88–89t
   cardiac agents, 83–84t
   central nervous system agents, 74–79t
   chemical and cellular physiology, 48t, 49–51, 49f,
     50f
   dermatologic agents, 99–100t
   dosage forms, 51–52t, 72, 73t
   drug interactions, 102
   drug misadventures, 72, 101, 102t
   endocrinologic agents, 81–82t
   eye, ear, nose, and throat agents, 79t
   gastroenterologic agents, 80–81t
   genitourinary agents, 87t
   importance of pharmacotherapy, 48
   nutritional agents, 100t
   oncolytic agents, 95–99t
   pathophysiology, 67–68
   pharmacodynamics, 71–72
   pharmacokinetics, 64f, 69–71, 69f
   physiology, 65
   renal agents, 86–87t
   respiratory agents, 80t
   vascular agents, 84–86t
Drug dosages, and body mass, 12
Drug Enforcement Administration (DEA)
   controlled substance regulations, 35, 36–38, 36t,
     37f
   DEA numbers, 37
   Form 222, 36, 37f, 189
   history of, 35
   storage of medications, 193
Drug interactions, 102
Drug levels, 71–72
Drug preparation by pharmacists, 4

Histamine-2 antagonists, 80t
Homeostasis, 67
Hormones, 98t
Household equivalents, 20–21, 20t
Humidity, and medication storage, 194
Hypnotics, 74t

I

J

K

L

M

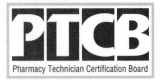

PTCB
Pharmacy Technician Certification Board

More than a test, it's the beginning of your career

PTCB National Pharmacy Technician Certification

National Standard for Excellence – The PTCB national certification and recertification program is the **only** pharmacy technician certification program to receive National Commission for Certifying Agencies (NCCA) accreditation. Join the over 270,000 pharmacy technicians certified by PTCB since 1995.

Testing Locations – PTCB delivers the Pharmacy Technician Certification Exam (PTCE) at more than 200 Pearson Professional Centers located throughout the United States and its territories allowing candidates to test at a location that is not only convenient, but also reduces travel time and expense. A complete list of test center locations is available at www.PTCB.org.

Testing Flexibility – The PTCB exam is administered during five-week testing periods, four times a year, giving candidates greater flexibility to take the exam at a time that best fits their schedule. Exams can be taken during the day and in some locations, in the evening and on weekends. With a wider choice of exam appointments and more testing locations, candidates have more flexibility and choice regarding when and where they test.

Registration and Scheduling – Registering and scheduling for PTCB exams is simple and flexible. Candidates have the ability to schedule and reschedule their exams up to 48 hours prior to the testing time without incurring additional charges.

Testing Experience – The Pearson Professional Centers are carefully controlled testing environments designed solely for high-stakes testing. The test centers are quiet, distraction free, and encourage peak performance from each candidate. With well-lit parking and easy accessibility from major highways, the test centers provide the best service, security and overall testing experience in the industry.

*Go to **www.ptcb.org** to register and schedule your test today.*